Basic Medicine for Emerg

Basic Medicine for Emergency Personnel

Roger Evans, MRCP,
Consultant in Accident and Emergency Medicine,
Cardiff Royal Infirmary

Patrick Durston, FASI,
Regional Ambulance Training Officer,
Trent Region

Butterworths
London · Boston · Durban · Singapore · Sydney · Toronto · Wellington

First published, 1985
Reprinted, 1987

British Library Cataloguing in Publication Data

Evans, Roger, *1942–*
    Basic medicine for emergency personnel.
    1. Medicine
    I. Title   II. Durston, Patrick
    610   R129

    ISBN 0–407–00314–2

Library of Congress Cataloging in Publication Data

Evans, Roger, MRCP
    Basic medicine for emergency personnel.

    Includes index.
    1. Emergency medicine.   2. Emergency medical personnel.
I. Durston, Patrick.   II. Title [DNLM: 1. Allied Health
Personnel.   2. Emergencies. WB 105 E92b] RC 86.7.E93
1985   616′.025   85–4237
ISBN 0–407–00314–2

Typeset by Phoenix Photosetting, Chatham, Kent
Printed and bound by Page Bros. Ltd, Norwich, Norfolk.

Preface

This volume is intended to provide some of the basic background knowledge which is needed by paramedical personnel, particularly those in the Ambulance Service.

It makes no pretence to cover the whole of anatomy, physiology medicine and surgery but is a précis, which it is hoped will aid the paramedic to understand the underlying disease processes in the patients who are being treated and transported.

We have tried to provide a solid foundation for those personnel who will wish to proceed to extended training using more detailed texts on specific subjects.

The authors wish to express their thanks to Christopher Hayne, FCSP for a major contribution to the Chapter on Patient Handling, and to Dr PSV Cox, OBE. for his substantial aid in preparing the chapter on Infectious Diseases. Also our gratitude must be extended to Janet Braddon and Barbara Durston whose secretarial services were invaluable and to John Newham for his advice and encouragement.

Contents

Chapter 1

Diagnosis and treatment

The human body functions like a complicated and sophisticated machine, and in health all its separate parts work closely together for their mutual benefit. The various parts of the body make up separate *systems*, each of which undertakes a different but linked task.

All the organs and structures which make up the body consist of millions of individual cells, and to keep these cells alive and to enable them to function properly a source of energy is needed. The energy is obtained from the food which we eat which is burnt inside the cells with oxygen from the air we breathe. However, for something like a slice of bread to be usable as an energy source by a cell, it has to be broken down, firstly into large starch molecules and then into much smaller sugar molecules. These minute sugar molecules are then small enough to be absorbed from the gut into the blood stream. This ingestion and subsequent digestion and absorption of food is the function of the gastrointestinal system (GIS).

The sugar molecules are absorbed from the gut and passed into the blood stream. Once in the blood stream they travel via the arteries and veins, 'pumped' along by the heart to wherever they are required, thus they are transported by the cardiovascular system (CVS).

When the sugar arrives at the cells, to act as an energy source, it is absorbed from the blood stream into the interior of the cells and there chemically 'burned' with oxygen producing energy and the waste gas, carbon dioxide. The oxygen has been transported from the lungs by the CVS, the respiratory system (RS) having extracted the oxygen from the air which is breathed into the lungs, and also, incidentally this system gets rid of the carbon dioxide by exhaling it.

Many other systems, e.g., the central nervous system (CNS) the urinary system (US), etc work together in the way we have just described, all functioning separately but inextricably linked together for the good of the whole. The complete failure of any one of these systems would result in the death of the patient.

1

Diseases

Inevitably throughout our life span we will fall victim to disorders of various sorts, some mild and transient, others severe and persistent, and still others fatal. For the sake of simplicity, diseases have been sub-divided into various groups and the major sub-divisions are:

(1) Congenital
(2) Acquired

Congenital

A congenital disorder is one with which you are born. This may be a minor blemish to the skin, e.g., a port wine stain, or a major internal defect such as a hole between the right and left sides of the heart.

Acquired

These are disorders which develop during the course of a patient's lifetime and are divided into several groups.

Idiopathic

These are disorders for which at present no underlying cause has been found, e.g., essential hypertension.

Infectious

These infections may be of any system, e.g., meningitis attacks the CNS, pneumonia the RS, and may be caused by one of several different types of organism, e.g., polio is caused by a virus, cystitis by bacteria, and athlete's foot by a fungus.

Degenerative

As the body ages so its various parts tend to deteriorate, some more quickly than others. For instance, sixty years of wear and tear on the cartilage in the knee joint can result in the degenerative disorder known as osteoarthritis.

Neoplastic

The term neoplasm means new growth and into this group come tumours of all types. Tumours may be benign in that they remain localized to their area of origin, do not invade surrounding tissues and if totally removed at operation they do not recur. Malignant tumours however, tend to invade other structures in their area of origin and also to spread widely (*metastasize*). Small pieces of the original tumour (the primary tumour) break off and are transported via blood vessels or lymphatic channels to distant parts of the body where they lodge and grow into secondary tumours, or metastases. Common sites for secondary tumours are in the lymph glands, the liver and the lungs but more or less any part of the body can be affected.

Malignant diseases of the blood such as acute lymphatic leukaemia, although they form no solid tumour are included in this group.

Traumatic

Trauma can produce damage which results in disease, for instance injury to the brain at birth can produce a child which is spastic.

Endocrine

Malfunctions of one of the endocrine glands of the body (*see* Chapter 13) can result in disease, e.g., a patient whose thyroid is not producing normal quantities of its hormone thyroxine, will suffer from the disorder myxoedema.

Autoimmune

Normally if a person becomes infected with a micro-organism such as the measles virus his body will be stimulated by the foreign protein of the virus to produce substances which destroy the invading organism. These substances are known as antibodies. Under certain abnormal conditions however, antibodies may be produced which attack not 'foreign' invaders but the body's own tissues producing what is known as an auto-immune disease, e.g., rheumatoid arthritis (RA) where antibodies attack certain parts of joints.

Iatrogenic

These disorders are brought on by the side effects of the therapy to a chronic pre-existing and unrelated disease. For instance, people with RA may sometimes be treated with one of the steroid anti-inflammatory drugs such as Prednisolone. Unfortunately, whilst this drug helps to reduce the inflammation in the joints afflicted by RA it also predisposes towards the formation of duodenal ulcers.

Disorders may be acute or chronic, acute diseases such as the bacterial infection of the bladder known as cystitis can occur out of the blue with the patient being well one day and the next experiencing severe burning pain every time they wish to pass urine. With appropriate antibiotic treatment the infection will be completely cleared within another 2 – 3 days, the whole event having occupied 4 – 5 days. Chronic diseases however, tend to linger on for long periods, months or years, or even for a lifetime. A chronic disease would be one such as asthma which can start in early childhood and may be present for the rest of the patient's life. Normally the condition will just grumble on in the background with the person on a minimum of treatment. Every so often, however it will flare up as an acute exacerbation and the patient will need extra therapy urgently to resolve this more severe episode.

Diagnosis

The diagnosis of a particular disorder is arrived at by:

(1) Taking the history of the illness;
(2) Examining the patient.
This tentative diagnosis is then confirmed by:
(3) Investigation.

The history

A history is obtained by talking to and directly questioning the patient, obtaining all the relevant details of his present illness and any information which may be important with regard to past illnesses and disorders which run in his family.

Examining the patient

The patient should be examined in an orderly fashion having a specific scheme in mind, for instance he may be examined one system at a time starting with his CVS, by checking his pulse for rate and rhythm, taking his blood pressure, etc and then having finished with that system going through all the others, e.g., RS, GIS, etc.

Investigations

There are very many sorts of investigations, some of which are cheap, easily performed, completely painless to the patient carrying no risk to life and which provide an almost immediate result. Such an investigation would be the testing of a patient's urine to see if it contains sugar.

At the other end of the spectrum would be an investigation like an endo-myocardial biopsy in which a fine tube (a cardiac catheter) is inserted into one of the main blood vessels in the groin and then pushed up into the heart. Once inside the heart a small piece of the heart muscle is cut away by a tiny pair of jaws situated in the tip of the catheter, and this tissue is then brought out as the catheter is removed. The tissue then has to be processed, cut into thin slices, stained and examined under the microscope before an answer is obtained. This investigation is expensive, requires great skill to perform, is uncomfortable for the patient as well as carrying a certain risk and no answer is available for 4 – 5 days.

Thus when investigations are being completed those that are easy, painless, cheap and quick are done first as if they provide confirmation of the diagnosis there is no point in continuing with the more painful and expensive investigations.

Tests on body fluids

These are carried out on blood, urine, sputum, etc. and the tests measure such things as the normal chemicals found in the fluids, e.g., sodium, potassium, etc and to check for the presence of any abnormal constituents, e.g., protein in urine, drugs in the blood, etc. The blood is obtained by venepuncture, i.e., inserting a hollow needle into a vein and drawing back a blood sample into the attached syringe.

Radiological tests

The use of X-rays has increased as more and more new techniques have been introduced to increase the number of structures which can be visualized and to improve the definition of the 'picture'. Straightforward, so-called *plain* X-rays only show up structures which are dense, e.g., bone. These structures are called *radio-opaque*. Most of the body is made up of structures which do not show up well on X-rays and are known as *radiolucent*. To visualize a radiolucent structure such as the stomach, that organ has to be coated with a dense substance that is itself radio-opaque, e.g., barium sulphate, and this type of investigation is known as a *contrast* study. Table 1.1 shows commonly performed contrast studies which are produced by introducing a radio-opaque dye into some part of the body which is itself radiolucent.

TABLE 1.1. Commonly performed contrast studies

Radio-opaque dye used	Part of the body outlined
Barium swallow	This outlines the oesophagus
Barium meal	This outlines the stomach and small intestine
Barium enema	This outlines the large intestine
Intravenous pyelogram	This outlines the kidneys, ureters and bladder
Cholecystogram	This outlines the gall bladder and bile ducts
Angiogram	This outlines the heart and blood vessels
Lymphangiogram	This outlines the lymph channels
Myelogram	This outlines the spinal canal
Arthrogram	This outlines the inside of the joints

Other investigations which are performed by the radiologists but which do not all make use of X-rays are the scans of various sorts.

Isotope scans   These are produced by giving the patient an injection of a radioactive isotope which will be deposited in abnormal areas, e.g., fracture sites in bones. These 'hot' areas then show up on special X-ray plates.

Ultrasound scans   These are produced by directing high-pitched sound waves into the patient and picking up the returning 'echo' waves, on a special receiver as they bounce back from the various structures they meet.

Computerized axial tomography (CAT) scans   These are produced by putting the information gained by X-raying a patient, through a specially programmed computer, which can then produce pictures from the information it receives to show up structures which are normally radiolucent.

Nuclear magnetic resonance (NMR) scans   These make use of magnetic fields rather than X-rays to produce pictures which show up soft tissues, e.g. the brain, as well as the normal radio-opaque bone.

Electrical tests

Certain structures, e.g., brain, heart muscle and skeletal muscle, produce minute electric currents which can be picked up, amplified and recorded on special paper. An electrocardiogram (ECG) is a recording of the electrical discharges of the heart and allows the detection of various disorders, e.g., a heart attack. Other electrical investigations include electroencephalograms (EEG) which demonstrate the electrical activity of the brain and electromyograms (EMG) which record the activity in the skeletal muscle.

Endoscopic investigations

An endoscope is an instrument which allows you to look into body cavities. It resembles a black tube of about 1 cm in diameter and may be of varying length. It has a light source at one end which allows you to illuminate the interior of a cavity you are inspecting.

A gastroscope allows you to examine the interior of the stomach, whilst a bronchoscope is used for inspecting the bronchi of both lungs, and a cystoscope is used to look inside the bladder.

If, when you are examining a hollow structure, you find something abnormal inside, the endoscope will usually have an attachment which allows you to remove a small piece of this tissue for later examination under the microscope. This sample is known as a *biopsy*.

Treatment

Having reached a diagnosis, appropriate therapy is then instituted and treatment may be medical or surgical.

Medical

Medical treatment relies on the use of various drugs such as antibiotics (which destroy bacteria), hypotensives (which lower blood pressure) antidepressants, analgesics (pain killers) etc. and also on radiotherapy (the treatment of tumours by radiation), physiotherapy etc.

Drugs may be administered in one of a variety of ways. Most commonly they are given orally, the drug being then absorbed into the blood stream from the gut. A minor variation of oral treatment is to allow the tablet to dissolve beneath the tongue and then be absorbed into the blood stream through the mucous membrane of the mouth. This is known as sublingual administration and is the route used for the treatment of angina with glyceryl trinitrate (GTN) tablets.

Suppositories, which are inserted into the rectum, contain a drug which is released as the suppository is dissolved, and the active substance is then absorbed into the blood stream via the mucous membrane of the rectum.

Some drugs are absorbed through the intact skin and these are held in place, for instance on the chest wall, by a plaster, the drug slowly making its way into the blood stream over 24 hours, e.g., glyceryl trinitrate.

Some drugs, however, e.g., insulin have to be given by injection as they are destroyed by the action of acid in the gut if they are taken orally. Other drugs may be taken orally or by injection but the latter route is used when for instance it is a matter of urgency to get the drug into the blood stream, e.g., to relieve pain, or alternatively if a patient is too ill to take oral medication.

Drugs given intravenously (i.v.) act fastest as they are put directly into the blood stream, whilst those given intramuscularly (i.m.) and subcutaneously (s.c.) still have to be absorbed from the tissues into blood vessels in the area.

Occasionally drugs are put directly into the cerebrospinal fluid (CSF) at lumbar puncture, the so-called intrathecal route. This is used for the treatment of such conditions as meningitis.

Surgical

Surgical treatment involves some invasive procedure which may be minor, e.g., removal of a small skin tumour, or major, e.g., tying off a bleeding artery inside the skull.

Chapter 2

The cardiovascular system

Anatomy and physiology

The cardiovascular system (CVS) is the transport system of the human body. It brings oxygen and nutrients to all the cells of the body and removes carbon dioxide and waste products which are then carried to the lungs and kidneys for removal.

The system consists of two pumps which, when joined together, make up the heart and which work side by side distributing blood throughout the body via a network of interlinked tubes, the blood vessels.

Anatomy of the heart

The heart is cone-shaped and is situated beneath the sternum or breast bone with its apex pointing towards the left. Normally it is about the size of a large orange and weighs 300 – 350 g. It sits inside a double envelope, the pericardium, which totally encloses and protects it.

The two pumps, a left-sided one and a right-sided one, each pump blood around a separate circulatory system. The right side pumps blood around the lungs, the so-called pulmonary circulation, whilst the left side pumps blood to the rest of the body, the systemic circulation. Because it is much harder to pump blood around the systemic circulation rather than just around the lungs alone, the left-sided pump is much thicker walled and more powerful than the right.

Each of the pumps has two separate chambers, (*see Figure 2.1.*) an upper thin-walled chamber which acts as a reservoir, the atrium, and a lower thick-walled muscular pumping chamber, the ventricle. The ventricles, by contracting, produce the pressure which pushes blood around the pulmonary and systemic circulations. The heart is more or less entirely made up of muscle, the myocardium. This has a smooth inner lining, the endocardium, and an outer coating, the epicardium (*see Figure 2.2.*).

Each pump has two valves which permit flow in only one direction. The site of these valves is illustrated in *Figure 2.1*. They are the tricuspid valve between the right atrium and the right ventricle, and the pulmonary valve at the exit of the right ventricle where it is joined to the pulmonary artery. Between the left atrium and the left ventricle lies the mitral valve and at the exit to the left ventricle, where it is joined to the aorta, is the aortic valve.

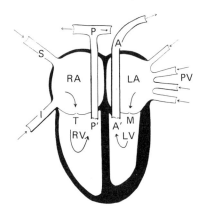

Figure 2.1 Diagrammatic representation of heart and major arteries: P = Pulmonary artery; P′ = Pulmonary valve; A = Aorta; A′ = Aortic valve; S = Superior Vena Cava; I = Inferior Vena Cava; PV = Pulmonary veins; RA = Right Atrium; LA = Left Atrium; T = Tricuspid valve; M = Mitral valve; RV = Right Ventricle; LV = Left Ventricle; Arrows indicate direction of blood flow.

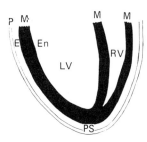

Figure 2.2 Diagrammatic representation of the heart as it lies within the Pericardial sac: P = Double layer of Pericardium; E = Epicardium (Outer surface of heart); En = Endocardium (Inner lining of heart); M = Myocardium (Heart muscle); LV = Left Ventricle; RV = Right Ventricle; PS = Pericardial Space.

Action of the heart

Although the two pumps operate synchronously, for the sake of simplicity we will just follow the blood on one circuit from start to finish.

Initially, 'stale' blood arrives at the right atrium (RA) via the inferior vena cava (IVC) from the lower half of the body and the superior vena cava (SVC) from the upper half of the body. This blood is a dark purplish-blue colour as it is full of the waste gas carbon dioxide which is dissolved in it.

When the RA is full the tricuspid valve opens and the muscle which makes up the wall of the RA contracts and squeezes blood out through the orifice into the right ventricle (RV). When the RV is full the tricuspid valve closes to prevent backflow of blood into the RA and then the muscular wall of the RV contracts, thus increasing the pressure inside the chamber and causing the pulmonary valve to open. Blood is thus forced up into the pulmonary artery (PA), and this blood is then distributed throughout the lungs.

Whilst it is in the capillaries of the pulmonary circulation close to the alveoli of the lung, it gives up the carbon dioxide it is carrying, and the gas passes into the alveoli to be breathed out. Meanwhile, oxygen from the 'fresh air' in the alveoli is absorbed by the blood and this 'freshened-up' blood returns via the pulmonary vein (PV) to the heart. The 'freshened-up' blood is now a bright pinky-red colour due to the oxygen it contains, and it re-enters the heart via the left atrium (LA).

The LA now begins to fill, and when full the mitral valve opens and the LA contracts and pushes the blood into the left ventricle (LV). When the LV is full, the mitral valve closes to prevent back-flow and the muscle of the LV starts to contract. The increase in pressure forces open the aortic valve and blood is pushed into the aorta under quite high pressure and starts on its journey around the systemic circulation.

When the fresh oxygen-enriched blood reaches an area which is working and therefore in need of oxygen, e.g., the thigh muscles of somebody who is walking, it gives up its oxygen which passes into the cells to form energy by burning with sugar. The waste carbon dioxide so formed now passes back into the blood stream and the blood consequently becomes dark purplish-blue in colour again. The flow continues back towards the heart, the blood eventually arriving once more in the RA, its trip through the two circulations now completed.

Contraction of the heart is sometimes known as cardiac *systole*, and the subsequent relaxation phase is known as *diastole*. These terms you will come across particularly in reference to the timing of murmurs.

The blood pressure

The head of pressure produced by the left side of the heart has to be sufficient to push blood right around the body from head to toe, and in a normal person reaches a maximum pressure of some 120 – 140 mm of mercury. It is known as the blood pressure and it is what a doctor measures when he pumps the inflatable cuff around a patient's arm and then listens with a stethoscope over the brachial artery whilst slowly releasing the pressure.

The blood pressure is measured by an instrument called a sphygmomanometer and we normally record it as two separate readings, e.g., 120/80. The first figure, known as the systolic pressure, is the highest pressure reached in the system whilst the second, or diastolic pressure, is the lowest figure to which the pressure in the blood vessels falls. the pressure varies, as when the pump on the left side of the heart contracts (i.e., ventricular systole) and ejects a spurt of blood, there is a rise in pressure, and then as the pump relaxes (i.e., ventricular diastole) and is refilled the pressure slowly falls until it is increased again by the next ventricular systole.

The pulse

As the wave of pressure produced by the ventricular systole proceeds along the arteries it can be felt as a pulse in the vessels. There are three main arteries that we use to check the pulse. These are the radial artery on the inside of the thumb side of the wrist, the carotid artery tucked in under the sternomastoid muscle in the neck and the femoral artery in the groin. You should make sure that you are adept in locating each of these pulses as an emergency is no time to find out that you are unaware exactly where they are situated. You should also know what a normal pulse feels like so that you can recognize an abnormal one when you come across it.

When you are checking a patient's pulse you should note the rate, normally 70–80 per minute in an adult but higher in children; the rhythm, normally regular in health and sometimes irregular in disease, and the volume – does the force of the beat of the pulse hit your fingers with a normal pressure or is it weak, 'thready' and difficult to locate?

Blood vessels

The blood travels around the body in a network of interconnected blood vessels. On leaving the left ventricle, blood enters the aorta and travels along it, this large vessel gives off various smaller arteries, e.g., the carotid artery to the head, and the brachial artery to the arm and blood is thus distributed around the body via these vessels (*see Figure 2.3.*). Arteries divide into smaller branches known as arterioles which then subdivide into the smallest of all blood vessels, the capillaries, which are of microscopic size. These vessels have walls which are very thin, so thin in fact that they will allow gases and nutrients to diffuse in and out of the capillary. In

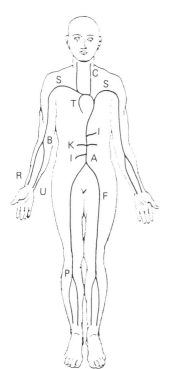

Figure 2.3 Diagrammatic representation of the major arteries: T = Thoracic Aorta; A = Abdominal Aorta; C = Carotid artery; S = Subclavian artery; B = Brachial artery; R = Radial artery; U = Ulnar artery; K = Renal artery; F = Femoral artery; P = Popliteal artery; I = Arteries to Intestines.

this way oxygen is allowed to leave the blood and pass into the cells of the various organs and tissues of the body whilst carbon dioxide and other wastes pass in the reverse direction into the blood vessel.

Groups of capillaries then gradually join together again to form larger vessels known as venules, several of these venules will then amalgamate to become a small vein and the veins will gradually rejoin to form a single large vein, the vena cava, which returns blood to the right side of the heart. Thus arteries take blood away from the heart, these subdivide to form arterioles and then capillaries which are thin-walled to allow the exchange of oxygen, carbon dioxide, nutrients and waste products. They then join together again eventually forming a vein which brings blood back into the heart. Arteries contain blood which is under much higher pressure that that in veins, they are therefore much thicker walled.

Coronary arteries

The heart itself, being an almost totally muscular organ which is working hard (it only gets short rest periods during diastole), needs oxygen and nutrients to keep it functioning properly. These are brought to it by the blood which gets to the myocardium via the coronary arteries, special blood vessels which run through the myocardium. The carbon dioxide and the waste products are returned to the right atrium via the coronary vein. There are two coronary arteries, the right and the left, and we shall discuss some of the problems arising in these important structures on page 17.

Investigation of cardiovascular disease

The two most important investigations in the emergency management of a patient with heart disease are:

(1) The electrocardiogram (ECG)
(2) The chest X-ray (CXR)

Electrocardiogram (ECG)

The ECG records the electrical currents produced by the heart muscle in its alternating phases of contraction (systole) and relaxation (diastole). Its main uses are in demonstrating damage to the myocardium such as occurs secondary to a heart attack (myocardial infarction), and also in aiding the precise diagnosis and treatment of abnormal rhythms of the heart (arrhythmias).

Chest X-ray (CXR)

The CXR will show us the size of the heart, demonstrating any enlargement, and also outline any abnormalities of that organ and of the great blood vessels leaving it (aorta and pulmonary artery). It will also give us some information with regard to the state of health of the lungs.

Other investigations

Later in the course of a patient's management other investigations may be undertaken. These include ultrasound and isotope scans and angiograms which are pictures of various parts of the heart and great vessels which are produced by injecting radio-opaque dyes and then X-raying the patient.

Examination of the heart

As well as checking the rate, rhythm, and volume of the pulse and the blood pressure, when the heart is examined clinically, great reliance is placed on the noises heard when a stethoscope is used to listen to the sound produced by the action of the heart. There are two major noises produced by the action of a normal heart. They are known as the first and second sounds and are caused by the mitral and tricuspid valves snapping shut simultaneously (first sound) and the synchronous closure of the aortic and pulmonary valves (second sound). The characteristics may change in a diseased heart and additional sounds and murmurs may appear. Normally, flow of blood through the heart and great vessels is smooth and noiseless, however, where flow becomes turbulent as when blood passes over diseased, distorted or leaking valves, a bruit or murmur appears and is audible via the stethoscope. Murmurs are classified as systolic or diastolic according to whether or not they occur during ventricular systole or diastole.

For instance, narrowing of the mitral valve (mitral stenosis) produces a diastolic murmur whereas leakage through an incompetent tricuspid valve (tricuspid regurgitation/incompetence) produces a systolic murmur.

Auscultation of the lungs can also be helpful as it may demonstrate a build up of fluid diffusely through the lungs (pulmonary oedema) or as a pool between the two layers of the pleura (a pleural effusion).

Other observable abnormalities which may occur in heart disease are swelling of the ankles (ankle oedema), a distension of the jugular vein in the neck (raised JVP) and sometimes cyanosis. Cyanosis is a blue/grey discolouration of the lips, cheeks and nail beds and is a sign of asphyxia as it demonstrates an excess of carbon dioxide in the blood together with a lack of oxygen.

Clinical features of cardiovascular disease

The commonest clinical features of cardiovascular disease are:

Chest pain

This is usually centrally placed behind the sternum and often radiates to the left shoulder and arm and up into the neck.

Shortness of breath (dyspnoea)

This can occur even at rest, indeed it is sometimes particularly severe at night and can come on suddenly (paroxysmal nocturnal dyspnoea) particularly if the patient slips down in the bed.

Patients with heart disorders often prefer to sleep in the semi-recumbent position propped up by four or five pillows, and the patient may be woken up suddenly if he has been lying flat for some time to find that he is gasping for breath.

Palpitations

This is an unpleasant awareness of the pumping action of the heart and is particularly noted when the heart is beating rapidly (a tachycardia).

Blackouts or dizzy/fainting attacks

These occur when the amount of blood pumped by the heart is inadequate to supply the brain with the oxygen it needs. It occurs if the heart is beating very rapidly or very slowly (a bradycardia) or occasionally where there is a narrowed heart valve e.g. aortic stenosis.

Specific cardiovascular disorders

Hypertension (high blood pressure)

Normally a healthy young person's blood pressure, as measured with a sphygmomanometer cuff at rest, is somewhere around 120/70 mm of mercury. Whilst it varies over any 24 hour period, being higher during episodes of strenuous activity and lower during sleep, should it become permanently elevated above a level of 150/95 the patient is said to be hypertensive. Levels such as these would be regarded as mildly hypertensive, a severe hypertensive might reach heights such as 270/200 or more. Mild to moderate hypertension has no specific symptoms related to it although patients with severe malignant hypertension often suffer badly with headaches and visual disturbances. The main signs and symptoms related to hypertension are those of the complications produced by the disorder. These complications include cardiac failure, renal failure, cerebrovascular accidents and myocardial infarction.

Hypertension may be caused by a variety of disorders such as diseases of the kidneys, tumours of the adrenal glands, or a narrowing of the artery taking blood to the kidneys (renal artery stenosis). However, in the majority of patients, no cause is apparent and the condition is known as *essential* hypertension. The condition is treated with drugs that lower the blood pressure, these are known as hypotensives and there are a wide variety of such compounds.

Commonly used are diuretics (drugs which increase the amount of urine produced) such as chlorthalidone (Hygroton) and amiloride (Moduretic), and Beta-blockers (drugs which sedate the heart) such as atenolol (Tenormin).

Ischaemic heart disease (IHD)

As discussed previously the myocardium needs a continuous supply of blood bringing it oxygen and nutrients via the coronary arteries. Under some circumstances a coronary artery becomes narrowed by fatty deposits (atheroma) and thus insufficient blood and hence oxygen is available for the particular piece of myocardium supplied by that artery. These areas of myocardium are said to be ischaemic (short of blood) or hypoxic (short of oxygen).

Angina pectoris

This is the chronic form of IHD and is usually manifested by central chest pain often described as tight or crushing, which sometimes radiates to the left shoulder/arm and/or throat and jaw. The pain characteristically comes on when the patient exerts himself, e.g., walking up a hill carrying a suitcase. The reason for the pain under these circumstances is that when the patient is exerting himself, all his muscles need more blood/oxygen to fuel them and therefore his heart has to pump harder and faster to get the extra blood around the body. As the heart has to work harder it also needs more oxygen/blood itself, where the coronary arteries are normal this increased demand for blood from the myocardium can easily be accommodated by increasing the flow rate. However, where there is narrowing of a section of one of the coronary arteries, blood flow cannot be so easily increased and the area of myocardium supplied by that particular vessel will become ischaemic and hypoxic. However, the heart cannot just stop beating so it continues to work even though part of it is ischaemic, and it is this ischaemic area which causes the pain of angina pectoris.

When the person feels the pain, his natural reaction is to stop climbing the hill, put his suitcase down and lean against a wall. Thus, by resting, he reduces the demands made by his body for oxygen/blood, this in turn relieves the heart of the need to pump so hard, and therefore the demand for oxygen by the myocardium itself is reduced to levels which can be coped with by the narrowed arteries. Under these circumstances therefore, the pain is relieved by rest. Other factors which can cause the heart rate to increase, e.g., anger and eating heavy meals, can also bring on angina.

The condition is treated by:

(1) Stopping the activity which produced the pain.
(2) Allowing a tablet of Glyceryl Trinitrate (GTN) to dissolve under the tongue.
(3) Sedating the heart with Beta-blockers which would prevent the heart rate from increasing excessively.

Myocardial infarction (MI) – (synonyms; heart attack, coronary thrombosis)

This is the acute form of IHD and occurs when a blood clot forms suddenly inside a coronary artery, often at a point where it is narrowed by atheroma. This sudden blockage cuts off the entire supply of blood to the area of myocardium fed by the blocked vessel and this piece of myocardium becomes *infarcted* i.e., it has died due to lack of oxygen.

The chief symptom of a myocardial infarct is severe crushing central chest pain which may radiate to the left arm/shoulder/jaw in the same way that the pain of angina does, but generally speaking the pain is much worse and is never relieved by rest.

The patient may be shocked and is sometimes short of breath due to acute pulmonary oedema. Almost invariably the rhythm of the patient's heart is disturbed and in the early stages there is a very high risk of ventricular fibrillation occurring. This results in the patient's death and indeed about 50 per cent of the patients who die with a heart attack do so suddenly before medical or paramedical aid reaches them. It is in the first 12–24 hours following the onset of their illness that patients are most at risk.

Treatment of an acute heart attack consists initially of administering pain killers (analgesics) such as morphine or heroin intravenously or intramuscularly, these drugs relieve the pain and the associated anxiety. If possible an intravenous infusion should be set up, running slowly, and the patient connected to a cardiac monitor in order that his heart rate and rhythm may be observed. Where it is available, oxygen should be administered to the patient through a mask.

If any arrhythmias occur, these will be treated with the appropriate anti-arrhythmic drug and any other complications such as cardiac failure will be treated as necessary. Should the patient suffer a cardiac arrest as he is at a high risk of doing soon after his heart attack, cardiopulmonary resuscitation (CPR) will be instituted until direct current (DC) counter-shock treatment of ventricular fibrillation is available.

The diagnosis of a myocardial infarction is confirmed by seeing characteristic changes on the ECG, and also analyzing the patient's blood. This latter test reveals high levels of certain substances known as cardiac enzymes which will have leaked into the blood from the cells in the dying piece of heart muscle.

Sometimes patients with IHD who suffer with severe angina which is unresponsive to drug treatment may have special X-rays known as coronary angiograms performed. These will show up any narrowing of the coronary arteries and if the block is a localized one, the patient may be operated upon and the blockage by-passed using a segment of a vein taken from the patient's leg (*See Figure 2.4*).

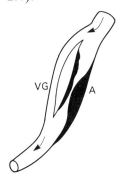

Figure 2.4 Segment of a coronary artery which is partially blocked by atheroma. The narrowed section has been by-passed by a short vein graft. A = Coronary Artery; VG = Vein Graft. The arrows represent the direction of flow of the blood.

Rheumatic heart disease (RHD)

The valves of the heart are made of a fine material with a consistency similar to that of the cloth of a nylon shirt. They are smooth, and the leaflets fit together perfectly only allowing blood flow in one direction.

The disorder known as rheumatic fever which usually occurs in children or adolescents can, in some cases, attack the heart valves and damage them, the result being that the valves become thick and distorted and the leaflets which made up the valve may be partially stuck together. A valve that is damaged may produce two functional abnormalities. It may be narrowed (stenosed, e.g., mitral stenosis – narrowing of the mitral valve), this stenosis impedes the flow of blood from one area to another. Alternatively, the valves may be leaky (incompetent, e.g., tricuspid incompetence – leaking of blood through the damaged tricuspid valve back from the right ventricle into the right atrium.) Both stenosis and incompetence may occur in the same valve, e.g., mixed mitral valve disease where the valve is narrowed and also leaky. If either or both of these abnormalities are present in a valve, it will of course impose an extra strain upon the heart, if the leak/narrowing is a minor one then the heart usually copes adequately. However, if the problem is more severe, the patient will gradually go into heart failure as its reserve strength is slowly used up.

The valves most commonly affected by RHD are the mitral and aortic, and the presence of the disorder is confirmed by auscultation of the heart and the detection of a heart murmur. Mitral valve disease is often accompanied by an abnormal rhythm of the heart, in which it beats irregularly. This is known as atrial fibrillation.

Congenital heart disease (CHD)

Whilst some people acquire damage to the valves of the heart following an attack of rheumatic fever others are unfortunate enough to be born with defects. Such people are said to have congenital heart disease and this may take a variety of forms. There may be narrowed or leaky valves or there may be holes in the walls between the right and left sides of the heart, e.g. atrial septal defect (ASD), a hole in the wall between the right and left atria, or a ventricular septal defect (VSD), an abnormal communication between the right and left ventricles.

Some patients are unfortunate enough to have multiple gross abnormalities of the heart which makes their survival unlikely. A few children with congenital heart disease may appear completely normal and the diagnosis may not be established until they are well into adult life. Others have severe disorders which result in them being cyanosed from birth, or they have disorders in other systems, for instance, children who are Mongols (Down's Syndrome) who have a characteristic facial appearance and are of low intelligence often have associated cardiac abnormalities. The abnormalities of CHD if severe will result in heart failure, the children being dyspnoeic even to the extent of being unable to feed due to having to gasp for breath continuously. They will often be undersized and may have a distended abdomen. They will need to be nursed/ transported in the semirecumbent position and will require treatment for cardiac failure in the usual fashion.

Arrhythmias

Normally a resting adult's heart beats regularly around 70 to 80 times a minute. This is known as sinus rhythm. If he exerts himself the heart rate will increase to supply his muscles with more oxygen, a sinus tachycardia, and when he is asleep his heart rate may well decrease, a sinus bradycardia. A child's heart rate will be higher than an adult's but it will still be regular. Any deviation from this regular rate when a patient is at rest is known as an arrhythmia. There are many different types, most of which need an ECG for their precise identification. If a patient's heart rate is more rapid than normal, say 120 per minute, he is said to have a tachycardia and if it is slower than normal, perhaps 50 per minute then this is known as a bradycardia (*See Figure 2.5*).

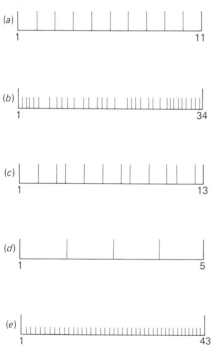

Figure 2.5 Diagrammatic representation of the characteristics of the pulse in various arrhythmias: (*a*) = Normal rate, rhythm regular (Sinus rhythm); (*b*) = Tachycardia, totally irregular, low volume (Atrial fibrillation); (*c*) = Normal rate, irregular rhythm. Extrasystoles (Beats 4, 8 and 11); (*d*) = Bradycardia, regular rhythm (Complete heart block); (*e*) = Tachycardia, regular rhythm, low volume 'thready' pulse. This type of pulse would be found in a 'shocked' patient.

Excessively fast rates put a great strain on the heart particularly if there is another underlying abnormality, e.g., ischaemic heart disease. It also means that the output of the heart can drop because there is too little time between beats for the ventricles to fill with blood. Patients with tachycardias often feel faint and unwell and they may complain of palpitations with a feeling that their heart is 'fluttering' inside their chest. A prolonged tachycardia may bring on heart failure or angina and precipitate the death of the patient.

Bradycardias may also precipitate heart failure or angina and can also produce dizzy turns and even black-outs which on occasions can be mistaken for epileptic attacks.

Tachycardias are usually controlled by the use of drugs given by injection, though occasionally the use of DC countershock is necessary. Bradycardias are also sometimes helped by the use of drugs but certain cases need to have a pacemaker inserted in order to increase the heart rate.

There are many different arrhythmias, however, we will only discuss five of the most important.

Atrial fibrillation (AF)

In this disorder the many muscle fibres forming the walls of the atria do not contract synchronously and this results in a tachycardia and a totally irregular heart beat. The condition is commonly found in rheumatic heart disease where the mitral valve is involved and sometimes in ischaemic heart disease. This rapid arrhythmia is treated using one of the digitalis group of drugs such as Digoxin and when the arrhythmia is controlled the pulse remains irregular but at a roughly normal rate.

Ventricular fibrillation (VF)

As in AF the muscle fibres which make up the ventricular muscle are not contracting in a co-ordinated fashion. The result is that no blood is ejected from the ventricles and the patient loses consciousness and will die if the rhythm is not corrected. Reversal back to sinus rhythm is attempted using DC countershock, the patient being kept alive by external cardiac massage until this facility is available.

Asystole

This, like VF, results in no out-put from the heart and consequent death. There is no cardiac activity at all and treatment consists of using drugs to induce some activity in the heart such as VF, and then hopefully shocking the patient back into sinus rhythm. All the while of course the patient is being kept alive by CPR.

Complete heart block

In this condition damage to part of the heart means that it can only run very slowly, usually no more than 40 beats per minute. These patients are prone to black-outs from which some of them do not recover. Treatment for this condition consists of connecting a pacemaker to the heart in order to keep it beating at a satisfactory rate.

Ectopic beats/extra systoles/ventricular premature contraction

Normal heart-beats originate at the top of the atrium in the sino-atrial node and work downward to end at the apex of the ventricles. This pathway ensures the most efficient action of the heart. However, under certain circumstances, for instance in the few hours following a myocardial infarct, extra beats may originate at sites other than the sino-atrial node and these cause an irregular pulse. They may arise from lower down in the atrium (atrial ectopics) or more dangerously from the ventricles (ventricular ectopics). Whilst atrial ectopics are benign and may be ignored, ventricular ectopics may disrupt the normal sinus rhythm and give rise to VF. These latter therefore need to be suppressed with drugs such as Lignocaine.

Heart failure

When the heart begins to fail and is unable to pump all the blood that it contains out of the ventricles into the great vessels (aorta and pulmonary artery), there is a build up in back pressure firstly in the atria and then in the great veins leading off them, i.e., the pulmonary vein and the superior and inferior venae cavae.

This back pressure is transmitted down the large veins eventually reaching the capillaries where fluid is forced out of the vessels into the tissues, this produces the boggy swelling around the ankles known as ankle oedema which is characteristic of heart failure. It will also produce a swelling of the liver which may be felt protruding abnormally from beneath the ribs on the right-hand side of the abdomen. When the back pressure rises in the pulmonary veins, fluid is extruded from the capillaries into the lungs and thus the patient starts to asphyxiate, as instead of air in his alveoli he has fluid. He is in effect drowning and thus people who are in heart failure are characteristically short of breath and have a chronic cough producing frothy white sputum sometimes tinged with blood. This is known as pulmonary oedema and can occur chronically or acutely as acute left ventricular failure (LVF), and the patient is agitated, gasping for breath, and cyanosed whilst coughing up lots of frothy sputum.

Patients who are in acute LVF with gross pulmonary oedema should be nursed and transported sitting upright with their legs dangling over the side of the bed. They should be given oxygen by mask and will benefit from a rapidly acting diuretic such as Bumetanide or Frusemide given intravenously, followed by morphine. Digoxin given orally is also used in patients with heart failure as it slows down the tachycardia where there is atrial fibrillation and strengthens the contractions of the failing heart.

Chapter 3

The respiratory system

Anatomy and physiology

It is via the respiratory system that the body is supplied with oxygen
and rids itself of carbon dioxide. Oxygen makes up roughly 20 per
cent of normal air whilst the remaining 80 per cent is made up prin-
cipally of nitrogen. This latter gas is inert and should concern us no
further.

Anatomy of the respiratory system

The respiratory system starts at the mouth and nostrils, these two
passages join to form the pharynx, the back of the throat, and this
then divides again in two, the oesophagus or gullet which carries
food to the gut and the trachea or wind pipe which takes air to the
lungs (*See Figure 3.1*).

Sitting on top of the trachea is the larynx which contains the vocal
cords, and just above the entrance to the larynx is the epiglottis, a
flap which can move up and down and which closes off the trachea

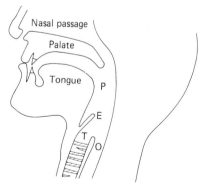

Figure 3.1 Longitudinal section through Head
and Neck: P = Pharynx; E = Epiglottis; T =
Trachea; O = Oesophagus.

25

when food is being swallowed, thus directing food down into the oesophagus and protecting the airway from blockage.

The lungs themselves have a spongy texture and sit inside the chest protected by the rib cage (thorax). They rest on the diaphragm, a thin sheet of muscle which separates the abdomen below from the thorax above. The lungs are enveloped by a double layer of membrane known as the pleura, in the same way that the heart is protected by the pericardium (*See Figure 3.2*).

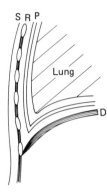

Figure 3.2 Diagrammatic representation of the structures making up the chest wall: S = Skin and subcutaneous tissue; R = Ribs connected by inter-costal muscles; P = The two layers of the pleura; D = Diaphragm.

The trachea divides into two branches, a left main bronchus and a right main bronchus supplying the respective lungs, the main bronchi then divide into several narrower segmental bronchi which in turn subdivide into smaller bronchioles (*See Figure 3.3*). The bronchi and bronchioles run right through the lung and end blindly as little balloons or air sacs which are known as alveoli.

The alveolus is very thin walled and has running around it a group of equally thin walled blood vessels, the microscopic capillaries. Because the walls between the air in the alveoli and the blood in the capillaries are so thin, gases can pass between air and blood quite easily and this is the site at which the gas exchange (oxygen from alveolus into capillary, carbon dioxide from capillary into alveolus) takes place (*See Figure 3.4*).

Mechanism of respiration

Air (20 per cent oxygen, 80 per cent nitrogen) is drawn into the trachea via the mouth and nostrils by an increase in the volume of the thorax. This takes place when the ribs move further apart due to the action of the intercostal muscles, and the diaphragm flattens.

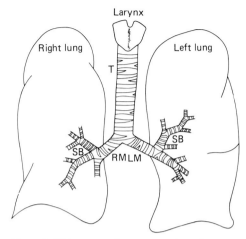

Figure 3.3 Diagrammatic representation of
Respiratory tree and lungs: T = Trachea; RM = Right
main bronchus; LM = Left main bronchus; SB =
Segmental bronchus.

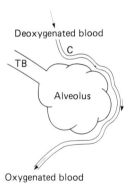

Figure 3.4 Diagrammatic representation of Terminal
Bronchiole and Alveolus surrounded by a Capillary:
TB = Terminal Bronchiole; C = Capillary.

Breathing out occurs when the diaphragm contracts and bulges
upwards and the ribs move closer together again. Air is thus
squeezed out of the spongy lungs and exhaled through the mouth
and nostrils. This is a straightforward bellows type of mechanism
and works well provided all the parts of the bellows are intact.
However, where multiple rib fractures occur, and the bellows
mechanism is disrupted, e.g., a flail chest, breathing can become
impossible.

Gas exchange

When fresh air is drawn into the alveolus it comes into close contact with blood full of carbon dioxide in the capillaries which surround the air sacs. Because the concentration of carbon dioxide is high in the blood and negligible in the alveolus, carbon dioxide tends to drift out of the capillary into the air sacs. With oxygen the situation is reversed, i.e., the concentration of oxygen is high in the alveolus and low in the blood, therefore oxygen drifts out of the air sac into the blood where it becomes attached to the haemoglobin in the red blood corpuscles. The oxygenated blood travels back to the left atrium, passes into the left ventricle, and is subsequently pumped around the body.

If carbon dioxide is dissolved in blood it gives the fluid a dark purplish-blue colour, whilst when blood has plenty of oxygen in it attached to haemoglobin, it is a bright pinky-red colour. Thus the blood that arrives at the alveolus from the right ventricle via the pulmonary artery is dark purplish-blue in colour (it is deoxygenated and full of carbon dioxide) and blood which leaves the alveolus bound for the left atrium via the pulmonary vein is pinky-red (oxygenated blood with no carbon dioxide).

The air which is breathed out of the alveolus is now made up of 80 per cent nitrogen, 16 per cent oxygen and 4 per cent carbon dioxide. One-fifth of the oxygen of the air therefore which was drawn into the lungs has been absorbed by the blood and replaced in the air in the alveolus by carbon dioxide which is exhaled.

The respiratory centre

The rate (15–20 per minute) and depth of breathing are controlled by the respiratory centre. This structure is situated at the base of the brain and constantly tests the blood which passes through it for oxygen and carbon dioxide. If the level of oxygen drops too low the respiratory centre increases the rate of breathing, and will similarly increase the respiratory rate if the carbon dioxide level gets too high.

Airway obstruction

Obstruction to the free passage of air between the nostrils and alveoli is a common, and usually avoidable, cause of death in patients who have an impairment in their level of consciousness. Normal people have reflexes known as the 'gag' and 'cough' reflexes which prevent the airway obstructing. For instance, when a foreign body touches the back of the pharynx in a conscious patient it tends to be coughed or vomited up, however, where a patient is unconscious these reflexes are inoperative and blood or vomit can accumulate in the back of the throat/mouth thus blocking the airway. Further, if the unconscious patient happens to be lying on his back there is a tendency for his tongue to sag in the back of his throat and again shut off the passage of air. Both of these problems can be avoided by putting the patient with an impairment of his conscious level in the recovery or coma position. If the patient has to be kept on his back, for instance where cardiopulmonary resuscitation is being undertaken, the airway may be kept open by extending the neck and supporting the head at the nape and the brow (*See Figure 3.5 a and b*), or alternatively by keeping the chin held forwards.

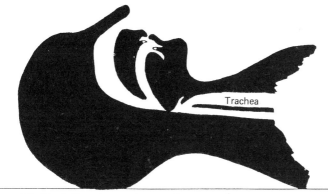

Figure 3.5a Head allowed to sag backwards. Tongue falls to back of throat blocking the airway.

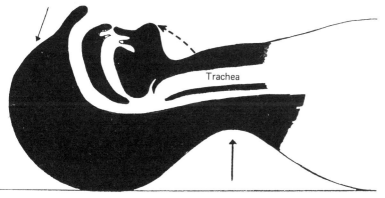

Figure 3.5b Neck extended by supporting head at nape of neck and brow (Force applied gently in the directions indicated by the solid arrows), or alternatively by keeping the chin held forwards (dotted arrow). The airway is thus kept open.

Clinical features of respiratory disease

Cough

The inner layer of the respiratory tract normally produces a slightly sticky solution known as mucus, which protects the delicate lining, and which also traps any dust or bacteria which are inhaled. This mucus is gradually brushed towards the mouth by the movement of fine hairs which sit on top of the cells of the inner lining of the lungs (these hairs are known as cilia). When the accumulated secretion reaches the back of the throat it is coughed up and thus the odd cough during the day producing grey-white sputum is quite normal. However, when the coughing is frequent, and where it produces sputum which is very sticky and difficult to cough up, or where the mucus is coloured yellow-green, i.e., it contains pus (purulent sputum) due to bacterial infection it must be looked upon as a symptom of disease. Occasionally also the sputum may be bloody (an haemoptysis) and this is an indication that bleeding has taken place into the respiratory tract (e.g. in carcinoma of the bronchus).

Shortness of breath (dyspnoea)

Whilst it is normal to be short of breath if you have run fifty yards to catch a bus, dyspnoea of this severity whilst you are sitting in an arm chair is certainly abnormal and is an indication of disease affecting the respiratory system. Dyspnoea also occurs in cardiovascular disease where this affects the lungs, e.g. pulmonary oedema.

Wheezing

A wheeze, heard particularly when patients are breathing out, is a common symptom of asthma and chronic obstructive airways disease. The wheeze is rather a musical sound and the patient often complains of his chest feeling 'tight' and that he is unable to get enough air into his chest.

Chest pain

The commonest form of chest pain associated with disease of the respiratory system is the so-called pleuritic pain. This pain may be localized to any part of the chest and is characteristically made worse by coughing and deep breathing. It is produced by inflammation of the pleura which can occur due to pleurisy or secondary to pneumonia, pulmonary embolism or rib fracture.

Stridor

This is a high-pitched noise heard on inspiration when the airway is partly obstructed high up in the region of the larynx/trachea.

Investigation of respiratory disease

The most useful investigation in the emergency management of patients with a respiratory disease is the chest X-ray. This will show us if the lung is properly expanded or even over expanded, it demonstrates tumours in the lungs, and infections such as pneumonia and tuberculosis. As well as this it will show up such things as fractured ribs, pleural effusions and enlargement of the heart.

Another useful test is to withdraw some blood from an artery (usually the femoral) and estimate the amount of oxygen and carbon dioxide in it, i.e., the blood gas levels. Where the lungs are failing the level of oxygen will drop and that of carbon dioxide will rise above normal.

Commonly people with chest infections have samples of their sputum taken and an attempt made to grow bacteria from this and then to test the sensitivity of the bacteria against various antibiotics.

A more invasive investigation often performed in units specializing in chest disease is bronchoscopy, where an endoscope is placed into the trachea and pushed down to inspect the main bronchi which are thus visualized and can be inspected for abnormalities, e.g., carcinoma of the bronchus.

There are several highly specialized tests of lung infection used in the management of respiratory disease but these have their place in the later management of such disorders.

Specific respiratory disorders

Pneumonia (Synonyms: pneumonitis, bronchopneumonia)

This is an inflammation of the lungs commonly caused by bacteria, but also sometimes due to viruses. It frequently follows a cold, and people who have chronic bronchitis are particularly prone to the disease. The elderly, and patients who are bed bound are another group who often suffer from pneumonia and indeed it can be a terminal event for geriatric patients. The complaint is often preceded by a cold and initially there is an abrupt rise in temperature up to 39 degrees C or more. The patient's breathing rate may increase, the breathing often being shallow and accompanied by a cough productive of purulent/blood streaked sputum. The cough, or attempts to breathe deeply may produce pleuritic chest pain and on inspection the patient may have cold sores (*Herpes labialis*, a virus infection) on his lips. He may look flushed, and on listening to his chest with a stethoscope it is often obvious that one area of his lung is clogged with purulent mucus and no air can be heard to enter that section. If he has pleuritic chest pain a pleural rub may be detected (a pleural rub is heard when the two layers of pleura are inflamed and rub against each other as the patient breathes in and out, producing a noise like two pieces of leather being rubbed together).

The diagnosis will be confirmed by a chest X-ray and the treatment will consist of 5–7 days of an appropriate antibiotic such as amoxicillin (Amoxil) or cephradine (Velosef). The patient is nursed in the semirecumbent position and he should be encouraged to cough up the infected mucus. Where necessary oxygen should be administered by mask usually at a concentration of no more than 24 per cent particularly where there is significant pre-existing chronic bronchitis.

Pleurisy and pleural effusion

Each lung is covered by two layers of a membrane known as the pleura, should the pleura become inflamed by bacterial infection for instance, the result is known as pleurisy. The commonest cause of inflammation of the pleura is pneumonia in the underlying lung though it also occurs secondary to pulmonary infarction and carcinoma of the bronchus. Pleurisy is manifested by the characteristic pleuritic chest pain which is accurately located at the site of the inflammation. The patient's breathing tends to be shallow due to the fact that deep breathing and coughing makes the pain worse. Pleurisy is treated by dealing with the underlying condition, e.g., treating the pneumonia with the appropriate antibiotics, though the pain of course is treated with analgesics. Sometimes fluid is exuded between the two layers of the pleura and it accumulates as a pool there. This is known as a pleural effusion (*see Figure* 3.6). Pleural effusions may arise from many causes, most commonly pneumonia/ pleurisy, congestive cardiac failure, and pulmonary infarction. A pleural effusion if large enough, and associated with other lung conditions, may cause a degree of dyspnoea, and when a stethoscope is placed over the affected area the normal breath sounds are barely audible. As with pleurisy, treatment is aimed at the underlying disorder, however, if the effusion is large and causing dyspnoea it may be necessary to insert a hollow needle into the pool and drain some fluid off.

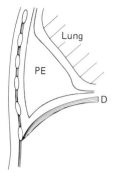

Figure 3.6 Diagrammatic representation of a Pleural Effusion: P = The two layers of the pleura; PE = Pleural Effusion; D = Diaphragm.

Asthma

This is a disorder which occurs intermittently and in which there are episodes of generalized obstruction of the airway caused by a spasmodic narrowing of the bronchi. It is characterized by dyspnoea often of acute onset and also a wheeze which is most marked on expiration. The patients usually have a recurrent cough which is productive of a very sticky mucus. The disease commonly starts in childhood and whilst it may last for the rest of the patient's life it is not unusual for it to disappear completely at around the age of 11 or 12 years. The underlying problem in asthma is the narrowing of the bronchi and this is mainly caused by two mechanisms. The first is a sustained spasm or contraction of the muscle in the wall of the bronchus (bronchospasm) which narrows the bronchus, whilst the second is the blockage of the bronchi by the sticky mucus which is very hard to cough up.

The characteristic history of an asthmatic patient is one of recurrent bouts of dyspnoea and wheezing lasting a day or two with episodes of normal respiration in between. The attacks may be brought on by an upper respiratory tract infection, e.g., a cold or sometimes by such things as violent exercise. There may be a history of asthma in the family or a past or family history of such conditions as eczema or hayfever. Asthma sufferers are often allergic to such things as pollen, housedust mites and the hair or fur of certain animals, and this allergy takes the form of constriction of the bronchi when these things are inhaled and drawn into the lungs.

The treatment of asthma consists of the administration of drugs which:

(1) Prevent the allergens acting on the bronchi and causing bronchospasm, these include inhaled drugs such as Disodium cromoglycate (Intal), and also steroids which are preferably

administered by an aerosol inhaler, e.g. beclomethasone diproprionate (Becotide), or occasionally if absolutely necessary, by tablet or injection, e.g., prednisolone.
(2) Cause the bronchial muscle to relax (bronchodilators) e.g., salbutamol (ventolin). These drugs may be administered by aerosol inhaler or by tablet.

When a severe acute asthmatic attack occurs the patient may need to be hospitalized if he does not respond to treatment at home with bronchodilators. In hospital he will be treated with such drugs as intravenous aminophylline and steroids given orally and intravenously. Any precipitating cause such as a chest infection would be treated with antibiotics and the patient given physiotherapy to the chest to clear it of secretions.

Pneumothorax

A pneumothorax means that there is air between the two layers of the pleura in the same way that there is fluid in this space when you have a pleural effusion. There are two main types, the spontaneous pneumothorax and one which occurs secondary to trauma, e.g., fractured ribs or a penetrating chest wound. The spontaneous type occurs more often in young men than any other group, usually due to a leakage of air from a small spontaneous rupture in the outer surface of the lung which causes the build up of air in the pleural space and the consequent deflation of the lung.

The occurrence of a spontaneous pneumothorax is marked by sudden chest pain often associated with dyspnoea, the severity of the shortness of breath is related to the underlying lung function. If a pneumothorax occurs in a fit young man the dyspnoea may be barely noticed, however, if the patient already has severe chronic bronchitis then acute life-threatening dyspnoea may occur. The diagnosis will be confirmed by a chest X-ray, and if the pneumothorax is a small one and the patient not disturbed by it, no treatment is necessary as the lung will re-expand satisfactorily on its own. However, should the leak be a large one a tube may have to be inserted into the chest cavity and the air drawn off to allow the lung to re-expand.

A pneumothorax may occur secondary to chest trauma when the jagged end of a broken rib can puncture the lung or alternatively following a penetrating chest wound, diagnosis and treatment would follow the same lines as for the spontaneous pneumothorax.

There is one type of pneumothorax which is rare but dangerous, this is the 'tension' pneumothorax, where air enters the pleural space, but because of perhaps the flap of a chest wound acting as a valve, the air cannot leave. This may occur in the so-called 'sucking' chest wound when air is drawn into the chest during inspiration but cannot leave it on expiration, hence the pressure builds up inside the thorax as more and more air is drawn in with each inhalation. The increase in pressure which then occurs causes kinking and obstruction to the passage of blood in and out of the heart via the great vessels and this finally results in the death of the patient. Immediate action is required to seal the wound and prevent more air entering the thorax, then if the situation is critical the air needs to be released, a wide bore needle may need to be inserted between the ribs, just below the clavicle, in order to relieve the pressure inside the thorax.

Pulmonary embolus (PE)

Sometimes a blood clot or thrombus can form in part of the cardio-vascular system such as one of the deep veins of the leg (a deep venous thrombosis or DVT). In this site it may produce no symp-toms at all until a part of it becomes detached and floats up the vein heading towards the right side of the heart. In its detached form this piece of thrombus is known as an embolus and eventually the embo-lus will reach the right atrium, pass into the right ventricle and head out in the pulmonary circulation where it finally lodges in a branch of the pulmonary artery as a pulmonary embolus. Pulmonary emboli may occur in three forms:

Multiple tiny emboli

These occur over a period of months or years and are symptomless until enough of them have blocked small branches of the pulmonary circulation to bring about failure of the right side of the heart.

Embolus of medium size

This will end up jamming in a medium sized branch of the pulmo-nary artery and producing pulmonary infarction, i.e., death of a segment of lung tissue. This type of embolus presents with pleuritic chest pain, haemoptysis and a tachycardia.

Massive pulmonary embolus

This is so large that it lodges in the main pulmonary artery as it leaves the right ventricle. Such emboli can cause the death of the patient within minutes.

Formation of a DVT occurs most frequently in patients who are elderly and who have been immobile in bed for an extended period. However they are not uncommon to younger people and turn up in young women after childbirth or in patients who have had abdominal operations, as well as in women taking the contraceptive pill. The treatment of a pulmonary embolus is to give the patient anticoagulant drugs which prevent further clotting of the blood. Initially Heparin is given intravenously and this is followed by oral Warfarin for the long term management of the patient. Where a massive pulmonary embolus has occurred and the patient survives long enough to reach hospital, drugs which actually dissolve the clots such as streptokinase may be administered intravenously. Patients who have sustained a massive pulmonary embolus can, whilst being transported to hospital, suffer a cardiac arrest and will need energetic CPR.

Chronic bronchitis

This is a very common disease in the United Kingdom and is characterized by a persistent productive cough which gradually worsens over the years and is later accompanied by dyspnoea and a tendency to recurrent chest infections. There is a striking relationship between chronic bronchitis and cigarette smoking and also, though to a lesser degree, with atmospheric pollution. Chronic bronchitis is also linked to a condition known as emphysema, in this latter disorder the lungs become over inflated and this causes some of the alveoli to burst and become useless for exchanging oxygen for carbon dioxide.

Normally these patients cough persistently and produce a lot of grey-white sputum. When they have a chest infection the sputum changes colour to yellow-green, (i.e. it becomes purulent) and the patient may develop pneumonia. Gradually, over a period of years, the bronchitis will worsen and the patient become more and more dyspnoeic with eventual right sided heart failure resulting.

Treatment of this disorder consists of giving up smoking, treating infections with antibiotics as soon as possible, and giving bronchodilator drugs to those patients who have an element of asthmatic wheezing in their condition. Patients who have had severe chronic bronchitis for a number of years tend to have a persistently higher than normal levels of carbon dioxide in their blood and lower than normal levels of oxygen. Under these circumstances it is dangerous to raise the level of oxygen in their blood to too high a level as they then cease to breathe properly. Therefore, although when they have a chest infection they may need oxygen, it should be administered at a concentration of no greater than 24 per cent, initially with a special mask such as a Ventimask. Drugs such as those of the opiate group (morphine and heroin) and the barbiturates should be avoided as they sedate the respiratory centre and thus reduce the effectiveness of the patient's respiration.

Carcinoma of the bronchus (synonym: lung cancer)

This is commonest malignant disease in men and its occurrence is strongly linked with cigarette smoking. Only 5 per cent of patients who develop the disease survive 5 years, as a tumour can grow to considerable size inside the chest without causing much in the way of symptoms and hence is often far advanced and widespread before the patient feels unwell enough to consult his doctor.

Common methods of presentation are with a persistent chest infection, an haemoptysis, or sometimes just with general debility and weight loss. Diagnosis is made by chest X-ray and also by bronchoscopy when the tumour in the bronchus may be visualized and a piece removed for study under the microscope. Curative treatment is only attempted in some 20 per cent of all patients and consists of removal of part, or all of a lung, sometimes in conjunction with radiotherapy and/or anticancer drugs. For the vast majority of patients the only available treatment is palliative radiotherapy together with the use of strong analgesics to ease pain.

Occupational lung disease

There are many lung disorders related to occupations, some are due to the accumulation in the lungs of mineral dust, e.g., coal workers pneumoconiosis, quarry workers silicosis, etc., whilst others occur secondary to an allergic reaction in the lungs from inhaled dust, e.g., farmer's lung. The most sinister group are those in which the inhaled substance gives rise to a malignancy such as occurs following the inhalation of asbestos fibres. In the first group there would be a slowly worsening dyspnoea together with a cough productive of sputum which is often stained with the inhaled dust. Allergic conditions such as farmer's lung often present with acute 'asthma' attacks, associated with a fever which occurs after exposure to the irritant (in this case mouldy hay). Asbestosis produces progressive dyspnoea and later malignant tumours may develop.

Tuberculosis (TB)

Tuberculosis is an infectious disease caused by *Mycobacterium tuberculosis* which frequently, but not exclusively, attacks the lungs. It is much more common in the developing world than in the more prosperous countries and is now only occasionally seen in the United Kingdom. It is a chronic disease which grumbles on over months and years, rather than an acute condition like pneumonia in which a patient feels well one day and can be quite ill two or three days later and fully recovered again ten days after that. A patient may have quite extensive disease present and yet complain of no particular symptoms. However, common clinical features are weight loss, debility, fever and cough sometimes with an haemoptysis. Treatment of tuberculosis is with drugs such as isoniazid and rifampicin and whereas antibiotics such as ampicillin would, to treat pneumonia, be given for a week or so, antituberculosis drugs will be administered for months. Because TB can be present for an extended period without giving rise to symptoms, relatives may be unknowingly in contact with an infected patient for months and hence may themselves contract the disease by the time the original patient has been diagnosed. Therefore it is essential that all 'contacts' be checked and X-rayed to prevent further outbreaks.

Chapter 4

Shock

The organs and tissues of the body depend for their well-being on a constant supply of oxygen. If there is a generalized reduction in the amount of blood and hence oxygen circulating around the body, then the organs and tissues become hypoxic and they cease to function properly. This results in the condition known as shock. The word is used very freely by lay people, for instance a patient who may have been involved in a minor accident is often said to be 'shocked'. Shaken and upset they may be, in shock they are not. Shock is a very serious condition which is strictly defined and has a mortality of up to 75 per cent.

Causes of shock

Hypovolaemic

This is due to fluid loss, e.g., bleeding from a severed artery or plasma loss from extensive burns. Here the mechanism is quite obvious, the loss of fluid leads to a reduction in the amount of blood available to carry oxygen around the body.

Cardiac

This is secondary to damage to the pump (the heart), e.g., myocardial infarction. In this case an MI may have destroyed a good deal of the left ventricular myocardium, and the amount of muscle left cannot generate sufficient pressure to circulate adequate amounts of blood.

Obstructive

Under these circumstances there is a major obstruction to the flow of blood somewhere in the circulatory system, e.g., a massive pulmonary embolus where a large blood clot has produced a major blockage in the main pulmonary artery, and hence only a trickle of blood gets through the lungs and arrives at the left side of the heart.

Distributive

This occurs when there is a relative loss of fluid from the circulatory system caused by pooling of the blood, e.g., following a very painful injury there may be a generalized dilatation of blood vessels and hence, grativationally mediated pooling of blood in the lower parts of the body with a consequent reduced return of blood to the heart for onward pumping.

Recognition of shock

The following clinical features may be present:

(1) An impairment of consciousness.
(2) A tachycardia.
(3) A reduced blood pressure.
(4) Pale, moist skin.
(5) Cyanosis.

Treatment of shock

The treatment of shock begins with an attempt to treat the underlying condition, e.g., in hypovolaemic shock due to blood loss from a lacerated limb, control of bleeding is vital. The next step aims at improving the supply of oxygen to the organs and tissues which are most sensitive to hypoxia, e.g., brain, kidney, etc. The supply of blood to these vital organs can be temporarily increased by tipping the patient head down or lying the patient flat and elevating the legs. Both of these methods rely on gravity to get as much blood as is available to the brain and kidneys, at the expense of the lower limbs, which can withstand hypoxia for much longer. Where available, oxygen should be administered by mask and the patient hospitalized forthwith. As soon as possible after admission, an intravenous infusion is started and appropriate therapy commenced, e.g., in a patient suffering from blood loss due to a bleeding duodenal ulcer, replacement of blood is essential. Operative intervention may be indicated later but this is best left until the patient's condition has improved and is stable.

Other measures which may be necessary include the administration of analgesics, antibiotics, or drugs which help cardiac output and raise blood pressure.

The treatment of shock must be aggressive and rapidly available if there is to be a reasonable chance of survival for the patient.

There may be complications secondary to the period of hypotension experienced by the shocked patient and they will manifest themselves later. These include brain damage of varying degrees and/or acute renal failure.

Chapter 5

Cardiopulmonary resuscitation

Cardiopulmonary resuscitation (CPR) is employed where the patient's heart has ceased to beat effectively, i.e., a cardiac arrest (CA) has occurred. As the heart has stopped beating, no blood is being pumped around the body and hence no oxygen is received by the organs and tissues. Under these circumstances the anoxic organs quickly cease to function, and if their blood and oxygen supply is not restored rapidly they will be irreparably damaged.

The organs which are most susceptible to oxygen lack are the brain and kidneys, indeed the former will degenerate permanently in 3–4 minutes if no oxygen reaches it.

Where a CA has occurred, perhaps secondary to a heart attack, one of two arrhythmias may be present. The first of these is known as asystole, in this condition there is absolutely no activity in the heart at all. The second is ventricular fibrillation (VF) which is described on page 22. Both of these arrhythmias are potentially reversible though VF more easily than asystole, the aim being to return the patient to sinus rhythm by appropriate drug and/or electrical treatment (defibrillation). Thus where a patient has suffered a CA, his life may be sustained by CPR, as this maintains a blood and oxygen supply, albeit a reduced one, to the vital organs until the correct treatment is available to restore the heart-beat.

Recognition of cardiac arrest

Where a CA has occurred the following physical signs may be noted:

(1) The patient is unconscious.
(2) No pulse is detectable.
(3) The patient is not breathing.
(4) The pupils are dilated and do not react to light.
(5) No heart sounds are audible.
(6) The patient is pale and cyanosed.

The techniques of CPR

Basic resuscitation technique

The basic resuscitation technique is the same whether one or two operators are present, though obviously it is much easier if two trained personnel are available. We will initially discuss the techniques and then finally detail how you would put them into practice depending upon whether one or two people are involved.

When a diagnosis of cardiac arrest has been reached, the following procedure should be rapidly instituted:

(1) The patient is laid down on a firm surface.
(2) Give the patient a single forceful blow over the lower sternum. Check again that the pulse is absent, if so continue the resuscitative procedure.
(3) The airway is cleared of any debris and kept open by maintaining the neck in extension supported at the nape of the neck and the brow. (*See Figure 3.5* page 29), or at the jaw and the brow.
(4) You should now take over the patient's breathing for him, this is done by using one of three techniques: mouth to mouth resuscitation; mouth to nose resuscitation or mouth to airway resuscitation.

Mouth to mouth resuscitation

With the patient's neck kept extended and the airway open, make a tight seal around his mouth with your lips pinch his nose closed and blow hard enough to see his chest rise. Give four or five quick deep breaths initially in order to flush the stale air out of the patient's lungs and then settle into a rhythm of between 12–15 breaths per minute.

Mouth to nose resuscitation

This is used where there have been injuries to the mouth/jaw making mouth to mouth resuscitation impractical.

Mouth to airway

This is used where a Brook airway is available. This is a clear perspex tube one end of which is inserted into the patient's mouth and which holds his tongue forward keeping the airway clear. The other end of the tube sticks out of the patient's mouth and it is into this free end that the operator blows to inflate the patient's lungs.

By ventilating the patient artificially you are getting 'fresh' air into his lungs and he is getting oxygen into his blood stream and getting rid of CO_2. If his heart is beating, the oxygen is being transported around the body, if not, you must take over the function of the heart and begin external cardiac massage. Therefore check the carotid or femoral pulse, and if the heart is not beating:

(5) Position the heel of your hand over the lower half of the sternum, (*Figure 5.1*) put your other hand on top of the first and, in

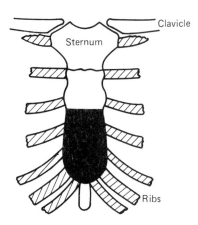

Figure 5.1 Diagram illustrating site of placement of hands for cardiac compression. The heel of one hand is placed over the lower half of the sternum, the other hand then resting on top of this. Site of compression is shaded.

an adult, depress the sternum sharply by about 5 cm (2 inches) (see *Figure 5.2*). Your arms should be held stiff and straight with the shoulders directly over the sternum, the downward movement should be smooth and there should be a short pause at the end of that stroke before pressure is relaxed and the sternum allowed to return to its normal position. This manoeuvre is repeated at a rate of about 60 compressions per minute, until the patient's heart restarts, or he is handed over to the hospital for continuing treatment.

The heart lies beneath the lower half of the sternum and in front of the vertebral column. When the sternum is depressed the heart is squeezed between it and the vertebrae and blood ejected. When the pressure is relaxed, the heart enlarges, drawing in more blood which is then pushed out of the heart with the next downward thrust. Thus a rather primitive kind of circulation is established which is about 30 per cent as effective as normal. Though this is far from ideal, it does get just enough oxygen around the body to keep the various organs alive until the patient arrives at hospital and attempts can be made to restart the heart.

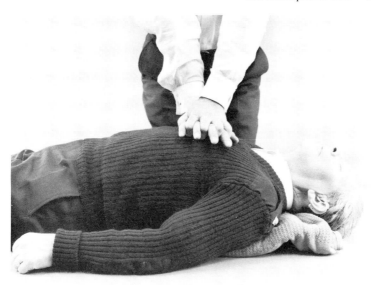

Figure 5.2 One method of positioning hands, with fingers linked.

If you are resuscitating alone, use the ratio of 15 compressions followed by 2 deep breaths into the patient's lungs, then a further 15 compressions and so on, i.e., a 15 compressions to 2 breaths ratio. If there are two resuscitators, quickly assign yourself to one of the jobs and begin working at a rate of 60 heart compressions per minute uninterrupted, the patient also getting a deep breath in the gap following each fifth compression, i.e., a 5 compressions to 1 breath ratio.

Some assessment as to the success of your resuscitative efforts may be judged by noting that the patient has 'pinked up' (i.e., he is no longer so pale and cyanosed), and that his pupils respond to light.

CPR in infants and children

The force with which you would blow to fill up an infant's or child's lungs is normally much lower than that for an adult, therefore modify your mouth to mouth technique appropriately. Also the child's neck does not need as much extending as an adult's and in fact, all that is necessary, is to lift the back of the child's head a little off the bed and support it on your hand or with a folded towel at the nape. Much less pressure is needed to depress the sternum and a fall of 2–4 cm (1–1½ inches) is usual. This may be achieved by quite light pressure with two or three fingers, or alternatively by wrapping both hands around the infant's chest, with your finger tips resting on the spine and your two thumbs over the sternum which then can be depressed gently. The compression rate for an infant or small child is 120 per minute, for a 5-year old 100 per minute and for older children 80 per minute.

Resuscitation in hospital

When the patient arrives at hospital, immediate treatment is instituted, this will take the form of the infusion of various drugs and fluids which correct the body chemistry and stimulate the heart. Sometimes in fact, these drugs will be given directly into the heart (an intracardiac injection). Defibrillation will also be necessary and this consists of the application of a direct current electric shock (DC countershock) across the heart from the base to its apex using a special machine (a defibrillator). The effect of the shock is to stop the heart, and hopefully, under favourable conditions, it will restart itself in sinus rhythm.

Use of a bag and mask

This is a manual resuscitator which is simple to use and consists of a self-refilling bag, a valve and a mask unit. Although it can be used in conjunction with an oxygen supply there is no dependence on any form of power so that it is immediately ready for use and light to carry.

After ascertaining that the patient is not breathing, place the patient in a supine position with a folded blanket under the shoulder blades in order to aid the tilt of the head and make sure that the airway is clear. Kneel behind the patient steadying his head between your knees, and then select the right size of mask. Place the mask over the patient's mouth and nose with the rounded edge placed on the chin and the pointed end over the bridge of the nose. Hold it in this position on the face by spreading the fingers of your hand so that the thumb is pressing down over the nose part of the mask and the index is over the chin part. Then spread your middle, ring and little fingers under the mandible lifting it upwards and forwards. When a good seal has been obtained the attached bag should be compressed, either by squeezing the bag with the fingers of the free hand or by compressing it against your thigh with your hand. When you release the pressure, the bag will refill and you should continue ventilating the patient as you would were you applying mouth to mouth ventilation. Do not forget to check the chest for a rise on inflation and a fall on deflation.

Mouth to mask technique

With yourself and the patient in the same position as previously described, place a cuffed mask over the nose and mouth, and whilst supporting the lower jaw with your fingers and maintaining an open airway, blow through the hole at the top of the mask to inflate the chest (*See Figure 5.3*). The advantage of this method over mouth to mouth or mouth to nose techniques is that it is easier for the operator and also that air will pass through both the mouth and the nasal passages.

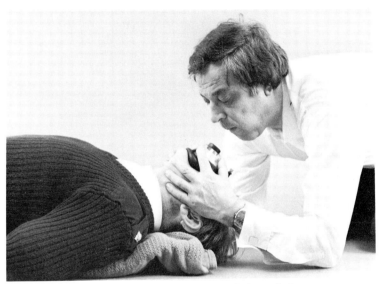

Figure 5.3 The mouth to mask technique of exhaled air ventilation.

Mouth to stoma resuscitation

Patients with a tracheostomy will have a small stoma tube sewn into the front part of the neck just below the Adam's apple. It will have the appearance of the top part of a pharyngeal airway. When the patient is breathing normally, inspiration and expiration is therefore through the stoma rather than through the mouth or nose. To resuscitate such a patient keep the head flat and do not hyperextend the neck, clear the stoma tube, close the patient's mouth and nose and then make a seal around the stoma with your mouth and blow directly into the tube.

The Holger–Nielsen technique

This is used as an alternative method of resuscitation for casualties who for instance may be trapped face down or who may have severe maxillofacial injuries.

(1) Place the patient in the prone position with his arms above his head, the elbows bent so that one hand is placed on top of the other under the patient's forehead, the head being turned to one side.

(2) Kneel (on one knee) at the patient's head with the other foot at the point of one of the patient's elbows. Place your hands palms down, one each side of the patient's thoracic spine just below

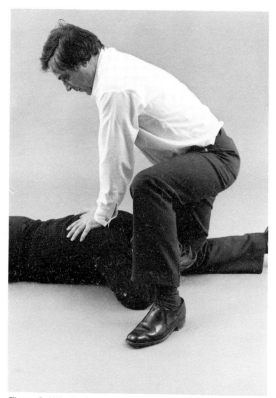

Figure 5.4 The Holger–Nielsen method of resuscitation. Air is being forced out of the lungs by steady pressure on the chest.

the shoulder blades, about 5 cm (2 inches) apart, keeping your arms straight and elbows locked.

(3) By rocking forward exert steady pressure on the chest for about 2 seconds (*see Figure 5.4*) then sliding your arms along the patient's chest and upwards and outwards along his arms, grasp the patient's elbows and pull them towards you until resistance is felt at the patient's shoulders (*see Figure 5.5*). This has resulted in air being drawn into the chest and should normally take about 3 seconds. The patient's arms are lowered and your hands replaced in their original position. This 5 second cycle should be repeated 12 times per minute.

(4) When the patient has recovered and breathing restarted, place him in the three-quarter prone position if possible, insert a pharyngeal airway and administer oxygen.

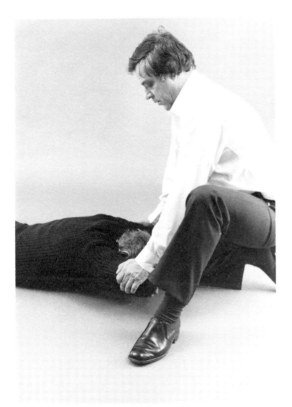

Figure 5.5 The Holger–Nielsen method of resuscitation. Air is now being drawn into the lungs.

The method is only practicable where there are no gross injuries to the arms, shoulders or thoracic cage.

The Sylvester–Brosche technique

This also is an alternative resuscitation method for patients with maxillofacial injuries.

(1) Clear the airway and keep it open.
(2) Kneel behind the patient supporting his head between your knees.
(3) Grasp the patient's forearms near the wrist (*see Figure 5.6*) and place them across the lower part of the chest.

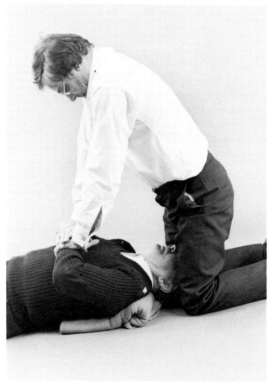

Figure 5.6 The Sylvester–Brosche technique of resuscitation. Air is being forced out of the lungs by steady pressure on the chest.

(4) Rock forward keeping your arms straight with your elbows locked and press down on the lower part of the chest wall for 2 seconds in order to expel air from the lungs.

(5) Draw the patient's arms upwards and outwards and backwards in a sweeping movement as far as they can go (reminiscent of rowing a boat), counting 3 seconds, in order to draw air back into the lungs (*see Figure 5.7*).

(6) Repeat the cycle every 5 seconds (12 times a minute).

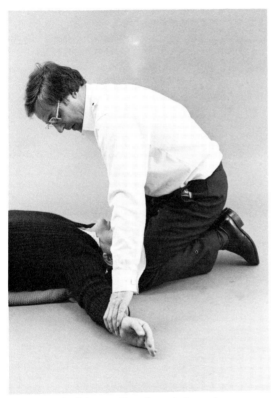

Figure 5.7 The Sylvester–Brosche technique of resuscitation. Air is now being drawn into the lungs.

Oxygen powered resuscitators

There are many types of such resuscitators on the market today, they should be simple to use, reliable and portable and should deliver oxygen at 100 *l* per minute with a pressure selection of 50 cm of water for an adult and 40 cm of water for a child, and be able to work off a D size cylinder.

Method

After ascertaining that breathing has ceased and that the airway is clear:

(1) Turn the cylinder on (usually four turns of a key), check the meter reading, press the button.
(2) Check that the setting on the head is correct, i.e. adult/child.
(3) Place the patient in the supine position, if possible with a blanket under the shoulder blades. Kneel behind the patient supporting his head between your knees.
(4) Select the correct size mask and fit it to the patient.
(5) With the airway clear and the jaw supported hold the mask lightly on the face, inflating the chest every 5 seconds by pressing the trigger. Only short bursts are required to inflate the chest and its rise and fall should be monitored continuously. Beware of pressing the button for too long as you may inflate the stomach, which is to be avoided as it obstructs the diaphragm and may cause vomiting.
(6) If the heart has stopped and cardiac massage is required simultaneously, the trigger will need to be pressed after every fifth compression.
(7) Upon recovery the patient is put into the three-quarter prone position with a pharyngeal airway inserted and oxygen administered.

Chapter 6

Haemopoietic system

Circulatory fluids

Under this heading we shall consider two closely related fluids, they are blood and lymph.

Blood

Blood consists of a fluid known as plasma in which are dissolved various salts and sugars and which has floating in it three types of cells: red blood cells (RBCs), white blood cells (WBCs) and platelets.

Blood transports all the substances necessary for the functioning of the organs and tissues of the body, for instance, sugar absorbed from the digested food in the gut is transported dissolved in plasma, whilst oxygen from the lungs is carried linked to haemoglobin in the RBCs.

The RBCs are full of an iron-containing protein called haemoglobin (Hb), a substance which has a natural affinity for oxygen. When Hb is exposed to high concentrations of oxygen, as it is when it is circulating in the capillaries around the alveoli in the lung, the gas becomes attached to the haemoglobin and is then transported around the body to reach an area which needs oxygen, e.g., the muscle of the leg. When the haemoglobin and oxygen reach such an area the gas is released and passes out of the capillary to the muscle cell.

White blood cells (WBCs) are far fewer in number than RBCs and their function is to keep the blood 'cleaned' and free from bacteria and other foreign material. They act as scavengers, consuming invaders, and also have a role in producing substances known as antibodies, these are proteins which fight infection in the body. There are two types of WBCs, first the myeloid cells (also called granulocytes) which are produced in the bone marrow and secondly the lymphoid cells (lymphocytes) which are also produced in the marrow, or alternatively in lymph nodes.

Platelets are much smaller than either RBCs or WBCs and their function is to assist in the clotting of blood. Blood coagulation depends upon an adequate number of platelets together with various chemical substances dissolved in the plasma known as clotting factors. These factors are all named and numbered, (e.g. Factor 1 fibrinogen, Factor 8 antihaemophilic globulin, etc), and for blood to clot properly all these clotting factors must be present in adequate amounts together with a sufficient number of platelets. When a blood vessel is cut and starts to bleed, a meshwork of sticky strands forms at the cut end of the vessel. These strands are made of a substance known as fibrin which is formed from Factor 1 (fibrinogen), but only when all the other clotting factors are available together with platelets. The strands trap red blood cells and thus form a blood clot which blocks the cut end of the vessel. If there are not enough platelets present (a condition known as thrombocytopaenia), or if one of the clotting factors is absent, (e.g. absence of Factor 8 antihaemophilic globulin, gives rise to the bleeding disorder haemophilia), then a blood clot will not form and the patient can bleed severely from a very minor wound. Platelets, like all RBCs and some WBCs are formed in the bone marrow, particularly in the marrow of the sternum and part of the pelvis.

Lymph

All the cells of the body are bathed in a fluid known as extracellular fluid (ECF), it is through this fluid that oxygen, carbon dioxide, nutrients (e.g., sugar) and waste products (urea) diffuse between capillaries and tissue cells. The ECF is being continually formed by diffusion of plasma fluid out of the capillaries and therefore also needs to be drained away in order to preserve a balance and ensure that the body does not become swollen by excess fluid (i.e., the body does not become oedematous). Drainage occurs into the lymphatic system which is an interlinked series of tubes similar to the blood vessels. The tubes often run alongside blood vessels and make their way towards the region of the heart and then drain into a large vein in the chest. They pass through various groups of lymph nodes which are situated at strategic points such as the axilla and groin, and these nodes filter out impurities such as bacteria so that when the lymphatic fluid enters the blood stream it is not infected.

Investigation of disease of the haemopoietic system

Blood can be easily studied by removing a sample from a vein, staining it, and examining it under the microscope. The formation of blood can be investigated by removing a sample of marrow from the sternum, again staining it and directly examining it under a microscope.

Clinical features of haemopoietic disorders

The commonest sign of a disorder of the haemopoietic system is pallor due to anaemia. The patient looks pale, and his conjunctivae (the inner surface of his eye lids) are also pale. Other common signs are lymphadenopathy (enlargement of the normally impalpable lymph nodes) and splenomegaly (enlargement of the spleen). A patient with a defect of blood coagulation may complain of being easily bruised and where the white blood cells are abnormal/ reduced in numbers, the patient will suffer frequent infections, as his body cannot combat an invasion by bacteria. The commonest symptom complained of will be weakness and lethargy.

Diseases of the haemopoietic and lymphatic systems

Anaemia

Anaemia is said to be present when there is a lower than normal amount of haemoglobin circulating in the blood stream. This disorder may arise for many reasons but there are four major types:

Iron deficiency anaemia (IDA)

This is the commonest type of anaemia and occurs when there is insufficient iron available in the diet to be incorporated with protein to produce haemoglobin. Iron is taken into the body in such things as meat, eggs, green vegetables and fruit, and is absorbed into the blood stream from the duodenum. It is then transported to the bone marrow where the protein part of the haemoglobin is produced, linked to the iron and packaged in RBCs.

Iron is of course also lost in small amounts from things like wounds, nose bleeds, and, in women, the monthly menstrual loss.

IDA will occur if the 1–2 mg of iron per day which is necessary to keep the body in balance is not available, due for instance to an inadequate diet.

IDA also occurs when, although the intake of iron is adequate for normal purposes, the patient is consistently losing blood, e.g., from a duodenal ulcer (DU) which is continuously oozing blood.

Under either of these circumstances when the body is not getting enough iron to cover the inevitable losses, IDA occurs. Whilst IDA can obviously be treated by improving the diet and by giving the patient oral iron supplements in the form of tablets, it is always important to check that the anaemia is not due to an excessive blood loss, e.g., from an oozing DU, rather than inadequate diet as it would be important to heal the DU rather than just treat the anaemia that it is causing.

Vitamin deficiency anaemia

Both vitamin B_{12} (cyanocobalamin) and folic acid are necessary for normal haemopoiesis (i.e., the formation of blood cells). Vitamin B_{12} is found in meat, liver, kidneys, etc, whilst folic acid occurs in fresh green vegetables, meats and cereals. Where either of these two substances is absent, or only present in markedly diminished amounts, RBCs are not formed properly and anaemia results. This disorder is sometimes known as macrocytic anaemia for not only are the RBCs fewer in number than usual, they are also much larger than the normal cells (*macro cytes* means large cells).

Such a vitamin deficiency anaemia may be treated by improving the diet and by administering supplements of missing vitamins. Folic acid can be given by mouth, but B_{12} has to be given by injection every 1–2 months.

Both IDA and macrocytic anaemia result in a patient who looks pale and feels tired. The patient may also complain of shortness of breath and palpitations.

Haemolytic anaemia

Under certain circumstances RBCs, which would normally have a life span of some 4 months, die prematurely. These RBCs rupture (haemolyse), usually because the haemoglobin they contain is abnormal, and they can, in very severe cases, rupture within a week or so of being formed. Under these circumstances, though the body steps up production of RBCs remarkably, it is still unable to keep up with the rate of haemolysis and the patient becomes anaemic. There are several different types of haemolytic anaemia and some of them are inherited, often on a racial basis. For instance, sickle cell anaemia is often found amongst the American Negro population, whilst thalassaemia is predominantly found in peoples from the Mediterranean, e.g., Greeks, Italians, etc.

People who have a haemolytic anaemia may, as well as exhibiting all the signs and symptoms of iron deficiency anaemia, also be jaundiced and have a large spleen which is easily palpable on examination of the abdomen.

Aplastic anaemia

A patient with aplastic anaemia has a disorder of the bone marrow which results in very few blood cells, RBCs, WBCs, platelets, being produced. This type of anaemia is obviously severe and frequently results in the death of the patient. It can arise spontaneously from no known cause, or it may be secondary to damage to the bone marrow caused by one of a variety of drugs or chemicals, e.g., the antibiotic chloramphenicol, or the antiarthritic drug sodium aurothiomalate (Myocrisin). In aplastic anaemia the patient is pale and tired because of the scarcity of RBCs, and as there are also fewer WBCs produced to fight infection, he is also prone to recurrent and persistent infections.

Further, the absence of platelets results in impaired blood clotting and hence the patient bruises easily and small wounds tend to bleed profusely.

The condition can, in some cases, be treated by bone marrow transplantation from a compatible, possibly related, donor.

Leukaemia

Leukaemia is a disease caused by the uncontrolled proliferation of WBCs. Normally there are some 8000 WBCs per cubic millimeter of blood and around 600 times as many RBCs. In leukaemia, the cells in the bone marrow which produce WBCs proliferate enormously. This has two consequences, first, the number of WBCs in the blood is grossly elevated and, secondly, the number of RBCs and platelets is reduced. As well as being present in high numbers up to 10–20 times the normal level, the WBCs are also abnormal and therefore ineffective in their task of fighting off invading organisms. In view of this the patient often presents with recurrent persistent infections, he lacks resistance to invading organisms, and he may be pale and lethargic (due to anaemia) and covered in bruises due to the low number of platelets.

Either one of the two types of WBCs (myeloid or lymphoid) can proliferate and may produce either an acute or a chronic leukaemia, e.g., acute lymphatic leukaemia (ALL), chronic lymphatic leukaemia (CLL), acute myeloid leukaemia (AML), etc.

In chronic leukaemias the patient usually survives 3–4 years from the time of diagnosis, whereas in acute leukaemias, if they are untreated, death will often result within a matter of weeks.

ALL tends to occur most commonly in children aged 3–5 years whilst AML is commonest in people over the age of 50. CLL and CML both tend to occur in patients in the 40 plus age group. The treatment of leukaemia aims to destroy the abnormal WBCs and thus allow RBCs, platelets and normal WBCs to be produced. Anticancer drugs are used and the patient is given blood and platelet-rich transfusions to support him whilst he is being treated.

Lymphomas

Lymphomas are malignant tumours of the lymph glands, there are several different types, the most well known being Hodgkin's disease. These disorders are characterized by a generalized enlargement of the lymph nodes, though these may increase and decrease in size. The liver and spleen may also enlarge and if lymphoma tissue infiltrates bone marrow the patient may become anaemic as the blood forming tissue is crowded out. The lymphomas are treated by radiotherapy and by chemotherapy with anticancer drugs.

Defects of blood coagulation

For blood to clot properly all the clotting factors and an adequate number of platelets must be available. Where one factor is absent blood does not clot properly and the patients bleed profusely from small wounds, and bruise easily and severely. Such conditions include haemophilia, an inherited disorder where there is an absence of factor 8, and Christmas disease where there is an absence of factor 9. Thrombocytopaenia, or a gross reduction in the number of platelets in the blood also produces failure of the clotting mechanism.

The treatment of disorders such as haemophilia and Christmas disease consist of the frequent and regular intravenous administration of the absent clotting factors.

Lymphangitis and lymphadenopathy

If you have a wound on the back of your hand which becomes infected by bacteria you may sometimes develop a tender red line underneath the skin which appears to be working its way up the arm from the infected wound. This occurs because the lymphatic vessel draining the area of the wound is taking away ECF which contains bacteria and this infected fluid causes the lymphatic vessels to become inflamed. This condition is known as lymphangitis. When the bacteria reach the lymph nodes in the axilla, these nodes swell up and become tender.

This swelling up of normally impalpable lymph nodes is known as lymphadenopathy and occurs not only in bacterial infections but also in infections due to other types of organisms and where the lymph nodes have become infiltrated with tumour cells, e.g., from carcinoma of the breast. If the lymphadenopathy is secondary to a bacterial infection, treatment with the appropriate antibiotic will result in the slow disappearance of both the lymphangitis and the lymphadenopathy.

Chapter 7

The central nervous system

Anatomy and physiology

The Central Nervous system is the command and communication system of the human body, and it can be divided into three parts:

(1) The Central Nervous System (CNS) made up of the brain and spinal cord.
(2) The Peripheral Nervous System, a network of nerves connecting the CNS with all other parts of the body.
(3) The Autonomic Nervous System which controls the automatic functions of the body.

The central nervous system (CNS)

The brain acts as the central control and is connected to all parts of the body by nerve fibres which run from the brain, down the spinal cord and outwards via the peripheral nerves. Messages travel as electrical impulses rapidly in both directions keeping the brain in touch with, and in control of, the peripheral parts of the body. The brain sits protected inside the skull and its extension, the spinal cord, leaves the base of the skull via a large hole, the foramen magnum. The cord runs down the back in the spinal canal, protected by the vertebrae, and giving off, at regular intervals, peripheral nerves which travel out to link all parts of the body with the brain.

The brain and spinal cord are surrounded by three membranes, the meninges, which help to protect it. The outer membrane is the tough leathery *dura* which is closely applied to the inside of the skull. The middle membrane is the *arachnoid*, and the inner one the *pia* which is very fine and is adherent to the brain and cord. Between the pia and arachnoid, is a space, the subarachnoid space, which is filled with a clear fluid known as cerebrospinal fluid (CSF). CSF is manufactured in small chambers inside the brain (the ventricles) and these chambers are connected to the subarachnoid space by narrow channels. It is via these channels that the CSF leaks out of the ventricles to surround and cushion the brain and spinal cord. Because of the close association between the brain and the CSF, certain diseases affecting the brain or meninges will produce changes in the CSF and thus the illness may be detected in a sample of fluid drawn off at lumbar puncture, where a needle is passed between the second and third lumbar vertebrae into the subarachnoid space.

The peripheral nerves are of two sorts, sensory (i.e. they pick up and transmit sensations such as heat, cold, pain, vibration etc) which carry messages to the brain, for instance that an object which is too hot has just been picked up. The other type are known as motor nerves and these carry instructions from the brain to the periphery, for instance to tell the muscles of the hand holding the hot object that they should relax and release the object allowing it to fall.

The brain consists of several distinct areas, the largest part is the cerebrum or cerebral cortex which receives messages from most of the sensory nerves, interprets them and institutes the appropriate responses via the motor nerves. It is divided into right and left hemispheres and is arranged in a series of folds or convolutions and divided into lobes which are named in relation to the bones of the skull which overlie them, e.g., frontal, parietal, temporal, etc, (see *Figure 7.1*). Centrally situated in each cerebral hemisphere is a ventricle and it is here that CSF is manufactured.

Situated beneath and behind the cerebrum is the cerebellum

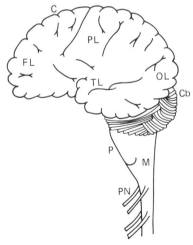

Figure 7.1 Diagrammatic representation of Brain and upper part of Spinal Cord: C = Cerebrum; FL = Frontal Lobe; PL = Parietal Lobe; TL = Temporal Lobe; OL = Occipital Lobe; Cb = Cerebellum; P = Pons; M = Medulla; PN = Peripheral nerves, the first two pairs leaving the spinal cord in the Cervical region.

which also receives a sensory input and has the function of co-ordinating movements and maintaining balance among other things. It also is divided into right and left lobes.

Lying in front of the cerebellum are the pons and the medulla, these two structures are the site of several of the body's most vital centres such as the respiratory centre (which controls respiration) and the vasomotor centre (which has some control over the cardio-vascular system).

Twelve pairs of cranial nerves arise from the brain and these serve various functions such as smell (the olfactory nerves), sight (the optic nerves), hearing (the auditory nerves), control of the muscles of facial expression (facial nerves) etc.

Structurally and functionally the brain is divided into two halves. However, it should be noted that the left side of the brain controls the functions of the right side of the body and vice versa. Therefore, damage to the right side of the brain produces a loss of function on the left side of the body.

The spinal cord commences at the foramen magnum and is a continuation of the medulla. It is about 46 cm (18 inches) long in an adult and extends to the level of the first lumbar vertebra. Like the brain it is protected by the meninges with CSF filling the space between the arachnoid and the pia. As the spinal cord runs down the back in the spinal canal protected by the vertebrae, it gives off consecutive pairs of nerves, one running to the left side of the body and the other to the right. These nerves run around the trunk and down the arms and legs and are called the peripheral nerves which keep the brain in touch with, and in control of, all the rest of the body.

The peripheral nervous system

Nerve cells consist of two parts: a cell body which is situated in the brain or spinal cord and a long 'tail' or axon which leaves the cell body to run down the spinal cord and out along the peripheral nerve, messages travelling up and down the axons as tiny electrical impulses. To facilitate the transmission of these electrical impulses many nerve fibres have a coating of a fatty substance (myelin) which acts as insulation. (*See Figure 7.2*). If an axon is severed, impulse transmission stops and regeneration of the axon, if it occurs, takes a very long time. If the cell body is damaged regeneration does not take place, unlike cells in other organs, e.g., the liver.

In summary then, the brain is constantly receiving information from the sensory nerves (e.g., sight, touch, hearing, etc) sorting that information, and then sending out instructions via the motor

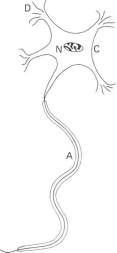

Figure 7.2 A single neurone or nerve cell. C = Cell body;
D = Dendrites, these maintain contact with adjacent
nerve cells; N = Nucleus; A = Axon, covered by its fatty
myelin sheath.

nerves to produce appropriate reactions to the incoming
information.

The autonomic nervous system

This part of the nervous system controls the automatic responses of
the body, i.e., it controls such things as heart rate and peristaltic
activity in the gut. The autonomic nervous system is made up of two
parts which often have opposing effects, these tending to balance
each other out. The two parts are known as the sympathetic and
parasympathetic systems and, for instance, whilst the action of the
sympathetic nervous system on the heart rate is to speed it up, the
parasympathetic slows it down. Thus, by both systems acting
together and keeping in balance, the heart rate runs at its normal
70–80 per minute when the patient is at rest. If a person is frightened

TABLE 7.1. Some effects of the two different parts of the autonomic system

Effects of sympathetic activity	Effects of parasympathetic activity
Increases heart rate	Decreases heart rate
Dilates bronchi	Constricts bronchi
Decreases motility of gut	Increases motility of gut
Dilates pupils	Constricts pupils

or threatened, the sympathetic nervous system increases its activity and the heart rate rises so that the person is 'ready for action'. The parasympathetic system conversely, would come into action where a person is relaxed and settling down to a large meal, under these circumstances the parasympathetic would be increasing the secretion of saliva and gastric juice to aid digestion.

Clinical features of central nervous system disease

The signs and symptoms of central nervous system disease as may be imagined can be many and various, the most common are discussed briefly below.

Impairment of consciousness

This may vary from a sudden complete permanent (up to the patient's death) loss of consciousness due to a major cerebrovascular accident (CVA or stroke) to the transient 'absences' seen in petit mal epilepsy.

Weakness (paresis) or complete inability to use (paralysis) a part of the body

This can vary from an almost undetectable weakness of part of the hand to complete paralysis of practically the whole body affecting even the muscles of speech and respiration.

Loss of sensation

This may be partial or complete, e.g., a total loss of vision in both eyes, or only loss of part of the visual field of one eye. It can include any of the types of sensation, e.g., hearing, touch, pain, etc.

Abnormal movements

Such as the tremors which occur in Parkinson's Disease.

Headache

This can occur and may be localized to one side of the head as in migraine or may involve the whole of the head. It is not uncommonly associated with nausea and vomiting.

Investigation of central nervous system disease

X-rays are the most useful tool in the investigation of CNS disease. Plain X-ray of the skull and vertebral column or the more sophisticated computerized axial tomography (CAT) or nuclear magnetic resonance (NMR) scans or ultrasound or isotope scans. Contrast studies such as carotid angiography (the injection of a dye, which shows up on X-ray, into the carotid artery, thus demonstrating the blood supply to the brain) or myelography (the injection of radio-opaque dye into the spinal canal to show up any points of narrowing such as might occur secondary to an intervertebral disc prolapse).

Outside the radiological field the most useful tests are the lumbar puncture which we have already described, and which measures the pressure of the CSF and allows a sample to be drawn off for analysis. This is a vital step in the diagnosis of infections of the CNS such as meningitis. The other group of investigations are the electrical ones, where the electrical activity of the brain, nerves and muscles is recorded as in an electroencephalogram (EEG), or an electro-myogram (EMG).

Specific neurological disorders

Cerebrovascular accident (CVA or stroke)

Any impairment of blood supply to the brain causes damage to that structure, the extent of the damage and its consequent effect on bodily function is related to the magnitude of the impairment. Thus a thrombus (a blood clot) forming in a small vessel in the area of the cerebrum controlling the function of the left hand may only cause some weakness and clumsiness in the hand, however a large haemorrhage from a ruptured cerebral blood vessel on the left side of the brain may cause total paralysis of the right side of the body and the death of the patient within a relatively short time.

The impairment of the blood supply is usually caused by the rupture of a weakened artery in the brain, this cuts off the blood supply to the area which is normally fed by that vessel, which then dies. Further damage is caused by blood leaking out of the artery and destroying tissue in the surrounding area. Other causes of CVAs include the formation of a blood clot in a cerebral vessel and also occasionally an embolus may lodge in one of the arteries inside the brain and thus block it. Such an embolus is usually a small part of a blood clot which has formed in another area of the CVS, e.g., a diseased part of the heart, a small piece of this clot breaks off and floats around in the blood vessels eventually lodging in a small artery.

Whether the CVA is caused by a haemorrhage, thrombosis or embolus, death of brain tissue results with consequent impairment of functions in the part of the body controlled by the damaged part of the brain. Whilst the extent of the symptoms and signs can vary from very minor, to major ones with death following shortly after, the usual picture is of an elderly patient who has perhaps, long-standing hypertension (hypertension predisposes to strokes later in life). The patient suddenly finds that he is unable to move the limbs on one side of his body properly and often finds his speech is slurred and that he cannot make himself understood. His face on the affected side may sag, and he finds that he is dribbling from the corner of his mouth. Alternatively the patient may suddenly lose consciousness and remain unconscious for several days, usually slowly recovering but finding that he is unable to use one side of his body.

The treatment of such cases in the immediate aftermath of the event consists of the protection of the airway from blockage by the sagging tongue and accumulated secretions, such patients who have an impairment of their conscious level must always be put in the recovery position. Longer term treatment consists of rehabilitative physiotherapy with the aim of improving the weakness (paresis) or overcoming the immobility (paralysis) of the limbs, and usually some improvement can be expected. Excessively high levels of blood pressure can be controlled with hypotensive drugs and in the few cases where an embolus was the cause, anti-coagulant drugs (e.g. Warfarin) will be indicated to prevent a recurrence.

Subarachnoid haemorrhage

This is a particular type of CVA where the vessel which ruptures is a relatively large one lying not in the substance of the brain itself, but in the subarachnoid space between the arachnoid and the pia. The patient presents with a severe headache of very sudden onset, lights hurt their eyes, and they feel pain and stiffness in their neck.

Epilepsy

There are several different types of epilepsy of which we shall consider two.

Petit mal (minor epilepsy)

In this condition there are repeated episodes of transient (2–3 seconds) loss of consciousness which result in the patient stopping whatever he is doing and appearing rather dazed. In these brief 'absences' the patient may appear to be staring into the distance and may look rather pale. When he 'comes to' he will carry on with whatever he was doing, often unaware that anything unusual has happened. Treatment consists of anticonvulsant drugs to prevent the attacks. Drugs used include ethosuximide, etc.

Grand mal (major epilepsy)

Major epilepsy manifests itself with rather dramatic convulsions, the following is the normal sequence of events:

(1) There is sometimes an initial period of irritability.
(2) Some patients experience an aura or strange feeling which warns them that an attack is imminent.
(3) Consciousness is lost abruptly and the patient falls to the floor sometimes injuring himself in the process.
(4) The rigid unconscious patient may be incontinent of urine and does not breathe.
(5) Spasms of the face, trunk and limbs may occur.
(6) The spasms are followed by short jerky movements when the tongue may be bitten.
(7) The movements gradually cease, the patient relaxes and becomes comatose.
(8) After 30–60 minutes, consciousness slowly returns though the patient may be confused and have a headache.

The treatment of the attack consists of trying to prevent the patient injuring himself first when he falls, and subsequently when he is on the floor jerking and possibly striking things such as an electric fire, or biting his tongue. An attempt should be made to put something like a tightly rolled handkerchief between his teeth in order to prevent the tongue being bitten. There is nothing to be gained from attempting to prevent the jerking movements. When the movements have stopped the unconscious patient should be put into the recovery position and any wounds sustained dealt with. The long term treatment consists of the use of anticonvulsant drugs such as phenytoin, clonazepam, and carbamazepine in dosages which are just sufficient to prevent the recurrence of convulsions. Strict rules must be applied about such things as driving and also about epileptics engaging in work under conditions which might be potentially dangerous, e.g., with unguarded machinery.

Febrile convulsions

The human body has a sophisticated control mechanism which keeps a healthy person's temperature fairly constant around 37 degrees C (98.4 degrees F). This system is not fully developed at birth and hence babies and infants are prone to develop marked fluctuations in temperature. An infection will cause a much higher rise in temperature in a baby than would occur in an adult who had a similar infection. This excessive and rapid rise in temperature can produce a 'fit' or febrile convulsion. Such events are common occurring in about 4 per cent of children and do not mean that the child will subsequently be an epileptic. They occur between the ages of about 6 months and 5 years though most commonly around 15–18 months.

The usual story is of a child who has been feverish and who suddenly rolls his eyes back and starts to twitch and jerk. The unconscious infant may not breath for a short time and may become cyanosed.

The child's airway must be protected and he should be given oxygen if available, the temperature is reduced by removing clothing and tepid sponging. If necessary anticonvulsant drugs may be given, and also antipyretics (drugs to reduce the temperature e.g., aspirin). If a bacterial infection is the cause of the disorder, antibiotics may well be necessary.

Hysterical fits

These occur as a reaction to a stressful situation and are not true convulsions. The patient will simulate what they think a 'fit' looks like, however, in doing so they will not hurt themselves, though as they often lash out wildly, they may well hurt bystanders and damage property.

Do not attempt to struggle with them, this will only exacerbate the situation. The more attention they get, the better will be the 'performance'. They are best treated calmly and are safest when allowed to lie on the floor in a darkened room under discreet observation, though occasionally they may need sedation.

Migraine

This is an episodic disorder which is characterized by a headache which can be very severe and which may be confined to one side of the head. It is often associated with visual disturbances, such as loss of a part of the patient's field of vision and sometimes by seeing coloured lights, etc. The patients often feel nauseated and may vomit and indeed can be totally incapacitated by the disorder. The disease is caused by contraction and dilatation of the arteries to the head, and is treated with analgesics and drugs which prevent spasm and dilatation of the arteries.

Meningitis

Meningitis occurs when an infective organism such as a bacterium or a virus gets into the CSF and inflames the meninges. About 80 per cent of cases are caused by viruses but the most dangerous type of meningitis is that caused by bacteria (*Neissera meningitides, Haemophilus influenzae, Mycobacterium tuberculosis*). The onset of the disease may be sudden, and the patient is febrile (feverish) with photophobia, neck stiffness and headache, which in severe cases may progress through drowsiness and coma to death. Some cases will also develop a rash.

Diagnosis is made by removing a sample of CSF at lumbar puncture and examining it. Normal CSF is clear and colourless but fluid removed from a patient with meningitis will be cloudy or even frankly purulent.

Viral meningitis is normally a benign condition from which the patient recovers satisfactorily with supportive care, however, bacterial meningitis requires aggressive treatment with the appropriate antibiotics. Close contacts of patients with meningitis due to *Neissera meningitides* sometimes require prophylactic antibiotic treatment as there is a possibility that they might themselves develop the disease.

Multiple sclerosis

This is a disorder of unknown cause in which the insulating, fatty, myelin sheaths which surround the axons of some nerves are destroyed, thus impairing the transmission of messages along those nerves. The patient usually presents with such symptoms as an impairment of vision of sudden onset, or of clumsiness, unsteadiness or perhaps weakness in the limbs. Characteristically the disorder runs a slow, downhill course with alternate relapses and remissions. After each relapse there is a good but not complete recovery and thus the patient is seen to be slowly deteriorating, getting a little worse after each relapse.

Gradually over perhaps 10 years the patient ends up in a wheelchair with some degree of incontinence, failing vision and slurred speech, later becoming bedbound with death resulting from an infection such as pneumonia. There is at present no cure for the disease though many different drugs and diets are used in an attempt to retard the progress of the disorder.

Intracranial tumour

Primary intracranial tumours are fairly rare in the population as a whole, they are however, relatively more common in children, arising most frequently in the region of the cerebellum.

Secondary tumours however also occur having spread via the blood stream from primaries in such situations as the bronchus and the breast.

Amongst those tumours that arise primarily in the brain about 50 per cent are malignant and 50 per cent are benign. The malignant tumours are only completely removable in exceedingly rare circumstances and hence treatment is palliative and consists of radiotherapy or chemotherapy. Unfortunately, many of the benign tumours also cannot be totally removed so that they recur and may subsequently cause the patient's death.

Tumours growing inside the closed box of the skull cause an increase in pressure inside that box and the consequent raised intracranial pressure manifests itself by the three classical symptoms of headache, nausea/vomiting, and drowsiness. Intracranial tumours may present in many other ways, e.g., convulsions, visual impairment, personality changes, inco-ordination, etc and because of this, diagnosis may be difficult and is best made by scanning the head, either CAT, NMR or isotope scans.

Encephalitis

This is an infection and inflammation of the actual substance of the brain and is predominantly a viral disease. The commonest virus causing this disorder in the United Kingdom is *Herpes simplex* which may cause an acute febrile illness with drowsiness and convulsions which may precede coma and death. The mortality rate is around 60 per cent as there are no satisfactory antiviral drugs presently available. Diagnosis is difficult and can only be made positively by identifying the virus in a sample of brain tissue obtained at biopsy. In other parts of the world, encephalitis is commonly a seasonal illness occurring in summer, as it is spread by mosquitos and ticks. Many of these summer fevers are much milder than *Herpes simplex* encephalitis and carry a much better prognosis.

Parkinson's disease

This is a disorder in which the patient finds it difficult to initiate movements, and even when he does so, the movements are slow, stiff and tremulous. The disease occurs most commonly in elderly men and is gradually progressive. The patient has a characteristically staring gaze and is immobile, apart from a persistent tremor, usually of the hands. When walking, the patient has a stiff, unsteady, shuffling gait. Drugs such as Levodopa are used to relieve some of the symptoms, however, they do not prevent the progression of the disease and the majority of patients are dead within 10 years of the onset.

Spina bifida

In this disorder which may vary widely in severity, the spinal cord, and the vertebrae which normally surround it do not form properly. The disorder may vary from a situation where a child is stillborn with its whole spinal cord lying open and unprotected along its back, to the baby born with the appearance of complete normality, having just a dimple at the base of its spine, and who has no neurological abnormalities or defects whatsoever (spina bifida occulta).

Many children with this disorder lie between these two extremes, they are born alive, and have some neurological impairment particularly affecting the legs (weakness or paralysis) and the sphincters of the bowel and bladder (resulting in incontinence of urine and faeces). Some surgical procedures are available to improve the quality of life of these children, however generally speaking they require special care throughout their lives. The condition is frequently associated with hydrocephalus.

Hydrocephalus

Cerebrospinal fluid (CSF) is manufactured inside the ventricles of the brain and normally escapes via three narrow channels to subsequently surround and protect the brain and spinal cord. In a child who is born with hydrocephalus these three channels are either completely or partially blocked which results in a build up in the amount of CSF inside the brain. This build up in turn causes the brain to enlarge and hence the head enlarges as the bones of the skull in an infant are not yet completely joined together, as they are in adults.

If the condition is not quickly diagnosed and treated the head becomes greatly enlarged, and damage to the brain will result in various degrees of intellectual impairment. Treatment consists of the insertion of a special valve (the Spitz–Holter Valve) which allows the drainage of excess CSF out of the ventricles into the jugular vein.

Polio

This infectious disease is due to a virus which attacks nerve cells situated in the spinal cord. Most patients suffer from little more than a mild influenza-like illness, however in some people, where the nervous system is attacked, paralysis of the limbs and more seriously the muscles of respiration and swallowing can occur. These are obviously life-threatening complications and death can result unless prompt treatment by tracheostomy and artificial ventilation is undertaken. The disease is prevented by the vaccination of infants.

Chapter 8
Unconsciousness

Unconsciousness is a sign that the activity of the brain is impaired. It can result from many causes, the most common of which are listed below:

(1) Fainting
(2) Poisoning, either accidental or deliberate (including alcohol)
(3) Head injuries
(4) Epilepsy
(5) As a complication of the treatment of diabetes
(6) Shock
(7) Hypothermia

Immediate treatment priorities

(1) Clear the airway and keep it open
(2) Arrest any haemorrhage
(3) Diagnose and treat any other injuries
(4) Keep the patient warm, dry and comfortable

The examination of the unconscious patient should be thorough and methodical so that no physical signs are missed.

You should not make assumptions, (e.g., that because a patient's breath smells of alcohol, that this is the cause of his unconsciousness) but make a proper assessment after considering all the facts. Make enquiries of relatives or bystanders, as you will need all the information you can get, in order to reach a diagnosis with a patient who is unable to answer questions.

For the accurate diagnosis of the cause of his unconsciousness, examination should always be carried out at skin level as many physical signs will be missed in the fully clothed patient.

Do not forget that many people carry on their persons cards, engraved bracelets (Medic-Alert bracelets), or lockets (Talisman lockets) which contain information which is often vital to their medical care, e.g., that they are diabetic or that they are epileptic.

Levels of consciousness

(1) Alert

The patient appears normal and answers questions accurately e.g., day of the week, time of the day, name and address, details of accident, etc.

(2) Confused or drowsy

The patient is drowsy often appearing lightly asleep and he has difficulty in orientating himself when woken. He may not be able to tell you exactly what happened and is often slightly confused.

(3) Stupor

He appears deeply asleep and will only respond to painful stimuli. He resents being woken but may be able to obey simple commands (e.g., to squeeze the examiner's finger). Any information forthcoming from him will be highly suspect as far as accuracy is concerned.

(4) Coma

He is deeply unconscious and cannot be roused even by painful stimuli, e.g., rubbing his sternum with your knuckles.

Examination

Having attended to the immediate priorities (airway, bleeding, etc.) talk to the patient and call him by name, if it is known. If you receive no reply apply minimal physical stimuli, e.g., tapping the cheek or pinching the lobe of the ear in an attempt to obtain some response so that you can assess his conscious level.

Note any odour on the breath, e.g., alcohol, or acetone (due to hyperglycaemic coma, page 128).

Inspect the mouth for injuries, e.g., broken teeth, bleeding from the tongue or inner surface of the cheeks. Do not forget that blood in the mouth may have been vomited up (haematemesis) from an internal bleed, e.g., from a duodenal ulcer.

Examine the lips for burns which might indicate that the patient has swallowed a corrosive poison.

At this point consider the insertion of a pharyngeal airway if one is available.

Next check the cervical spine for injury using the flat of the hand, feeling for abnormal lumps or any change in the shape and curve of the neck. If no injuries are suspected gently turn the head to one side.

External haemorrhage is not always visible through the clothing so quickly run your hands over and under the body checking for sticky dampness and immediately attending to any bleeding site located.

Check the pulse making a note of its rate, rhythm and volume, also check the skin and mucous membranes. Note if the skin is moist and covered with a fine perspiration as in shock, or does the patient appear pale or cyanosed, or perhaps warm, flushed and feverish.

The eyes

When examining the eyes check:

(1) The pupils. Are the pupils equal in size and do they both enlarge equally when shaded and diminish in size when a light is shone into them? Are these changes in size carried out briskly or sluggishly? Abnormalities of pupil size and reaction may occur secondary to bleeding into the skull or brain damage following severe head injury.
(2) The sclera (whites of the eyes). Are these blood-shot or perhaps yellow in colour (jaundiced)?
(3) The position of the eyes. Are they in a normal position or are they upturned, or deviated to one side as occurs in certain types of stroke?

The nose

Check for external injuries and also for bleeding or leakage of CSF, as may occur when the patient has fractured the base of his skull. (*See Figure 8.1*)'

The ears

Look in both ears for bleeding, the blood possibly mixed with CSF, or perhaps CSF alone. Both these findings might indicate a base of skull fracture. In addition place the small finger into the ear to feel

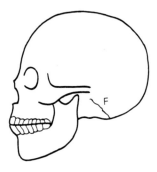

Figure 8.1 Diagrammatic representation of
base of skull fracture: F = Fracture line.

for dampness as it is sometimes difficult to detect the CSF by sight
alone.

The skull

Check for injuries visually, then starting at the forehead run your
hands through the hair, around the back of the head to the lower
jaw and facial bones, checking for abnormalities such as depress-
ions, swelling, bruising and bleeding. Take particular care with
movement especially if the history suggests the possibility of a spinal
injury. Check the lower jaw for movement and displacement in a
forward or backward direction.

The shoulder area

Check the bony structures in the area for fractures or dislocations
and examine the patient for wounds, particular attention should be
given to the neck and shoulder areas if serious head or chest injuries
are suspected. Check around the neck for a Talisman locket.

Chest area

Examine the rib cage including the sternum for fractures and watch
for abnormal movements whilst the patient is respiring, such as
might occur in a flail chest. Look for bruising which could indicate
damage to underlying structures such as the ribs, liver, lungs or
spleen and note any surgical emphysema (air having escaped from a
punctured lung and now lying under the skin). This can be heard
and felt when running the hands over the chest area, it sounds rather
like the crackling of tin foil. Do not forget to examine the back of
the chest.

Abdomen

Examine both front and back for wounds, bruising, extruded organs, or guarding (tensed abdominal muscles protecting damaged intra-abdominal structures), in which the abdomen feels board-like under the examining hand.

Upper limbs

Examine the whole of each limb separately and compare them, feeling hand over hand down the line of the bones starting at the shoulder. Check the brachial and radial pulses and the colour of the skin and nail beds. Examine the fleshy parts of the arms for puncture marks which are often present in mainlining addicts, then check all the joints for free movement.

The spine

Examine the whole of the spinal column, palpating the structure noting any abnormalities. Then if possible check it visually.

The pelvis

Examine the groin for dampness secondary to urinary incontinence as occurs in epilepsy, then check the bones of the girdle for any lack of rigidity.

Lower limbs

These should be checked in the same way as the upper limbs.

Finally re-check the level of consciousness, the patency of the airway, the pulse and the respiration.

Check through the personal effects for Medic-Alert cards, etc and for means of identification.

Check the patient's immediate surrounding area for drugs or any other clues which may be available.

Treatment

All unconscious patients except those with suspected spinal injuries should be placed in the three-quarter prone (recovery) position (*see Figure 8.2*) after examination has been completed and the injuries treated.

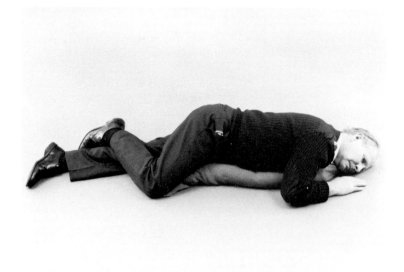

Figure 8.2 The three-quarters prone position, (recovery or coma position) with a coma roll in place.

Make sure the airway is kept open and never attempt to give the patient who has an impairment of consciousness anything by mouth, also do not forget never to leave them unattended.

Regular checks should be made on the level of consciousness, airway, respiration, pulse and pupil reaction. Note any changes in the condition of the casualty as an observation report would be helpful for the Accident and Emergency Department.

Observation report

A good observation report should include the following information:

(1) The type and time of the occurrence and a history of the incident.
(2) Your time of arrival at the incident and the condition of the casualty on arrival.
(3) The position of the casualty when first seen.
(4) The respiration and pulse rate.
(5) Any airway problems and how you dealt with them. A list of

any special equipment you used (airway, resuscitators, aspirators, etc).

(6) Any serious haemorrhage and how it was dealt with, together with an estimate of blood loss at the scene, en route, or on discarded clothing, and dressings.

(7) The level of consciousness and any changes (lightening or deepening, lucid intervals) and the total duration of unconsciousness.

(8) Pulse rate, rhythm, volume, times taken and any changes.

(9) Any leakage from the nose, mouth or ears.

(10) Any incontinence.

(11) Any other useful evidence such as cards, tablets, etc. and in the case of motorcycle incidents the crash helmet.

Chapter 9

The gastrointestinal tract

Anatomy and physiology

Food is necessary for the body, to act as a source of energy. However, before it can be used as a fuel, it has to travel from the mouth into the intestine and there be broken down into small enough particles to be absorbed from the gut into the blood stream. This breaking down of food and its subsequent absorption is the function of the gastrointestinal tract (GIT).

The GIT starts at the mouth, here food such as a starch in the form of bread begins to be broken down by being chewed and mixed with saliva. The lump of chewed food, now slimy due to being coated with saliva, is swallowed and slides down the oesophagus or gullet into the stomach.

The stomach churns up these lumps of food as they arrive and mixes the starch with diluted hydrochloric acid which is secreted by the stomach itself. The acid breaks the food down further and then the stomach passes it on into the first part of the small intestine, the duodenum.

Here again, the food is mixed with secretions from the pancreas, liver and the small intestine itself, which help to finally reduce the starch down to the minute size necessary for absorption into the blood stream as a form of sugar (*see Figure 9.1*).

The reduction in size is carried out not only by mechanical means (i.e., chewing and churning) but also by chemical means. Substances known as enzymes such as amylase are produced by the glands associated with the gastrointestinal tract, (e.g., salivary glands, pancreas, etc) they chemically split up the large starch molecules, which are too big to be absorbed by the gut, into their tiny constituent sugar molecules which are easily absorbed. Enzymes work similarly to break down other constituents of food such as proteins.

The absorption of the small sugars, which have resulted from the breaking down of the starch, takes place in the second part of the small intestine, the jejunum, together with all the other necessary

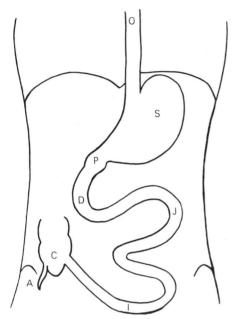

Figure 9.1 Diagrammatic representation of the
oesophagus, stomach and small intestine: O =
Oesophagus; S = Stomach; P = Pylorus. Small
intestine – D = Duodenum; J = Jejunum, and I =
Ileum. Part of Large intestine – C = Caecum and
A = Appendix

nutrients, which are totally absorbed by the time the contents of the
gut have passed through the third part of the small intestine, the
ileum. The remainder, the waste, passes into the large intestine.
  The first part of the large intestine is the caecum which lies in the
right iliac fossa. Leading off the caecum is the longest part of the
large intestine, the colon, which is divided into three parts,
ascending, transverse and descending, the final part leading on to
the rectum. There is a small blind-ending tube, the appendix, which
comes off the caecum and has no function in the digestion of food in
the human, however, it sometimes becomes blocked and
inflamed, producing appendicitis which may necessitate its
removal. The colon and rectum absorb any remaining water from
the gut contents and compact it into faeces which are passed to the
exterior through the anus (*see Figure 9.2*).
  The gut, apart from mouth, pharynx and oesophagus, lies almost
entirely inside the abdominal cavity which it shares with such organs

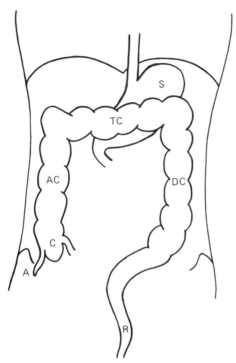

Figure 9.2 Diagrammatic representation of the large
intestine: S = Stomach; C = Caecum; A = Appendix;
AC = Ascending Colon; TC = Transverse Colon;
DC = Descending Colon; R = Rectum.

as the liver, kidney and pancreas. The cavity is lined with a membrane, the peritoneum, which surrounds the gut in the same way
that the heart is surrounded by the pericardium. The abdominal
cavity is separated from the thoracic cavity (chest) above, by a flat
sheet of muscle known as the diaphragm. The small intestine is
much longer (length 7 m, 22 feet) than the large intestine (length
2 m, 6 feet) but is called the small intestine as it is a good deal
narrower.

Food is moved along the gut by co-ordinated waves of muscular
contraction and relaxation which start in the stomach and move in
the direction of the rectum. This movement is known as peristalsis
and is an automatic function which is under the control of the
autonomic nervous system. A lump of food, which is swallowed at
the mouth enters the stomach via the oesophagus and then is gradually pushed along the intestine by the contraction of the muscle in

the gut in the area immediately behind it. As it is being pushed towards the rectum it is gradually being broken down and the nutrients absorbed from it.

Clinical features of gastrointestinal disease

The commonest symptom of gastrointestinal disease is abdominal pain. This, when it arises from a gut problem, is generally initially sited centrally in the abdomen though later it may move to localize over the site of the structure involved, e.g., the right iliac fossa in appendicitis. Abdominal pain may be present at the same level of severity continuously or may wax and wane in intensity (colic).

Other common symptoms of gastrointestinal disease are nausea and vomiting, the vomit usually being partly digested food from the stomach or sometimes blood (a haematemesis). Constipation or diarrhoea may also occur and blood may also be passed per rectum.

When an abdomen is examined, lumps or masses may be noted related to particular structures, e.g., a mass may be felt in the left hypochondrium (*see Figure 9.3*) produced by a carcinoma of the stomach, the organ which lies in that area. Normally when the muscles of the anterior abdominal wall are relaxed the abdomen should feel soft and be easy to examine. However, where there is an inflammation of the peritoneum, e.g., peritonitis, due perhaps to a burst

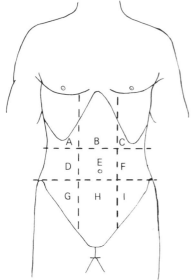

Figure 9.3 The subdivisions of the abdominal cavity: A = Right Hypochondrium; B = Epigastrium; C = Left Hypochondrium; D = Right Lumbar; E = Umbilical; F = Left Lumbar; G = Right Iliac Fossa; H = Supra-pubic; I = Left Iliac Fossa.

appendix or perforated duodenal ulcer, the anterior abdominal wall is held rigid and feels like a wooden board underneath the hand.

Investigation of gastrointestinal disease

The most useful investigations of gastrointestinal tract function are radiological and endoscopic. A straightforward plain X-ray of the abdomen is sometimes useful where there is obstrucion to the passage of food through the gut. However, more information is generally gained by the additional use of solutions of barium. A solution of barium, if swallowed, fills the gut and outlines it, as barium is radio-opaque, i.e., it shows up on an X-ray whereas the gut itself does not. Thus where a lesion is suspected in the oesophagus, stomach or small intestine, barium is swallowed (a Barium Meal), the lesion is thus coated with barium and shows up on X-ray pictures taken at the time. Where the disorder is situated in the rectum or colon, a tube is inserted into the rectum and barium injected (a Barium Enema), this outlines any disease in the large bowel. Endoscopes are special instruments which permit you to see into the body cavity and even to remove a small piece of tissue (a biopsy) which can later be examined under the microscope. They are used a great deal in the diagnosis of disorders of the gastrointestinal tract, i.e., a gastroscope might be used to inspect the inside of the stomach and remove a small piece of carcinoma which might be visualized, whilst a colonoscope would be used to view the inside of the large intestine.

Three important gastrointestinal problems

Before we go on to discuss specific disorders of the gastrointestinal tract, we will first deal with three problems related to gastrointestinal tract function which may be caused by many of the disorders we will subsequently consider.

Perforation

A perforation of the gut is said to have occurred when, for instance, a peptic ulcer burrows so deeply into the wall of the duodenum that it gradually works its way right through that structure. The hole so produced releases into the peritoneal cavity some of the contents of the gut which will contain very irritant substances, e.g., hydrochloric acid, often together with bacteria. These then attack the peritoneum and cause it to become inflamed, producing peritonitis. A patient who has perforated part of his gut usually has severe acute abdominal pain, and on examination the anterior abdominal wall is tense with all the muscles contracted and the abdomen feels rigid and board-like. A plain X-ray of the abdomen may show gas, which has leaked from the bowel, in the peritoneal cavity tucked up underneath the diaphragm. Treatment consists of repair of the perforation together with antibiotic therapy to combat the bacteria which have been released. Perforations do not occur only secondary to duodenal ulcers but may occur also with a malignancy anywhere in the gut, or in Crohn's disease, ulcerative colitis or appendicitis.

Obstruction

Under certain conditions the bowel may become obstructed and the passage of food through the tube is stopped. This results in abdominal pain, vomiting, distention of the abdomen and, once the segment of gut beyond the block has emptied itself, in absolute constipation as no more of the gut contents can get through. X-rays of the abdomen characteristically show loops of gut dilated with gas and fluids. Treatment is by surgical relief of the obstruction. Obstruction can occur secondary to hernias, tumours or such inflammatory conditions as Crohn's disease.

Gastrointestinal tract haemorrhage

Bleeding can occur from any site in the gut, when it is high up in the tract, e.g., oesophagus, stomach, duodenum, it may manifest itself as a haematemesis (the vomiting up of blood) or by the passage of black, sticky motions (melaena) which are made up of blood which has undergone digestion in its passage through the gut. Sometimes if blood remains in the stomach for a significant length of time it is attacked and partly digested by the hydrochloric acid secreted there and if subsequently vomited up resembles coffee grounds, as a dark brown granular substance.

Bleeding from lower down the tract, e.g., ascending colon, often presents as dark red jelly-like clots in the motions whilst bleeding from the rectum is usually in the form of bright red blood. Treatment of any significant degree of bleeding from the gut consists of replacement of the lost fluid via an intravenous infusion, followed by the identification of the bleeding site and sometimes surgical intervention to stop the bleeding if it does not arrest itself spontaneously.

Specific disorders

The oesophagus

Hiatus hernia

In this condition, which is very common, and in the vast majority of cases, quite mild, a part of the stomach has herniated (pushed its way through) the small hole in the diaphragm via which the oesophagus passes into the abdominal cavity. This herniation of a small part of the stomach, which is now up in the thoracic cavity most frequently results in the symptom known as 'heart burn', a burning pain in the chest and throat which is caused by regurgitation of the acid contents of the stomach up into the oesophagus. Hiatus hernia is common during pregnancy and as well as heart burn, can occasionally give rise to a more severe pain in the chest which can be difficult to differentiate from a heart attack. If the regurgitation of acid up into the oesophagus is severe and persistent, ulceration may occur at the lower end of that structure and this can result in bleeding, which sometimes manifests itself as a haematemesis. People with an hiatus hernia are generally more comfortable sitting well propped up rather than lying flat, as when they are flat there is likely to be more regurgitation up into the oesophagus. The treatment of the disorder is usually with a preparation, such as ranitidine (Zantac) or cimetidine (Tagamet), both of which prevent secretion of acid from the stomach. Other preparations used include all the standard 'white medicines' which are antacids (anti-acids) such as magnesium trisilcate (Mist. Mag. Trisil), or aluminium hydroxide which neutralize acid once it has been secreted.

Oesophageal varices

Under certain conditions, such as those which for instance exist in cirrhosis of the liver, the flow of blood through the liver becomes partly obstructed and this means that the veins that run towards the area, experience an increase in pressure and become dilated and tortuous. These varicosities as they are known, bear a superficial resemblance to the varicose veins frequently seen in the legs and in conditions such as cirrhosis, these dilatations often develop in the veins in the wall of the oesophagus.

   Such dilated veins bleed easily and freely and as patients who suffer from liver disease do not clot their blood as well as normal people, a quite severe haematemesis can result. These patients will often have signs and symptoms of liver cell failure and if they have recently bled acutely will be pale, covered in perspiration, with a rapid pulse and low blood pressure. Where such an acute bleed has taken place, the patient should be nursed head down with the legs raised, and have an intravenous infusion started as soon as possible in order to replace the blood they have lost. Care should be taken that they do not block their airway with vomit or blood.

When in hospital, energetic action should be taken to reduce and stop the blood loss as well as replacing the lost fluid. Drugs such as Vasopressin are administered intravenously, to reduce the amount of blood getting to the varicosities and in some cases an inflatable rubber tube is passed into the oesophagus and then blown up, thus compressing the dilated veins and hopefully stopping the bleeding. Further surgical procedures such as injecting the veins in order to cause them to clot (thrombose) are often undertaken later.

Peptic ulceration

The secretions produced by the stomach and small intestine (hydrochloric acid and various enzymes, e.g., pepsin) are intended to break down food. However, as they are good at their job they can also attack the lining of the stomach and small intestine, which therefore has to be specially protected against them. Occasionally this protection to the lining of the stomach or the duodenum breaks down and the juices secreted by the stomach act on these structures producing a peptic ulcer. If the ulcer is situated in the stomach it is known as a gastric ulcer (GU) and if in the duodenum, a duodenal ulcer (DU) results, the latter being about four times as common as the former.

The major complaint of ulcer patients is of a gnawing epigastric pain, particularly before a meal. The pain may be relieved by food, milk or antacids, such as Mist. Mag. Trisil., Andursil, etc. and these drugs are sometimes found in the bedrooms of such patients as the pain often occurs at night.

Diagnosis of these conditions is made by a Barium Meal and/or endoscopy, following which, treatment is via the use of drugs which block the secretion of acid, such as ranitidine (Zantac) or cimetidine (Tagamet). Occasionally an operation is necessary, most commonly, a vagotomy, where the nerve to the stomach (the vagus nerve) which controls the secretion of the acid is severed. Only rarely now is the operation of partial gastrectomy (removal of part of the stomach) necessary.

The two major complications of peptic ulceration are:

(1) Bleeding, where the ulcer penetrates a blood vessel, resulting in a haematemesis and melaena.

(2) Perforation, where the ulcer bores right through the wall of the gut and results in a leakage of the gut contents into the abdominal cavity.

Hernias

A hernia is said to occur when part of an organ, e.g., the gut, slips through a weak area of the wall of the cavity which normally contains it. For instance, part of the small intestine can bulge through the anterior abdominal wall at the umbilicus, producing an *umbilical* hernia (*see Figure 9.4*).

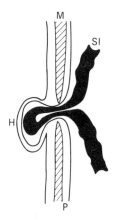

Figure 9.4 Diagrammatic representation of a hernia: H = Hernial sac containing a small piece of intestine, bulging through the anterior abdominal wall; M = Muscle of anterior abdominal wall; P = Peritoneum; SI = Small intestine.

There are several potential weak spots in the abdominal cavity and these are illustrated in *Figure 9.5*. The commonest sites for external hernias are in the groins where inguinal hernias occur.

A hernia, for instance, an inguinal one in the groin, usually presents as a soft swelling which initially may come and go, but which soon becomes established as a permanent lump which may be noticed to be slowly enlarging.

Such inguinal hernias are far more common in men than in women and the patient often realizes that he can, by gently manipulating the lump, push the contents back into the abdominal cavity and thus make the swelling disappear (i.e., they *reduce* the hernia). Hernias which are easily reducible are generally painless and indeed pain usually only occurs when complications set in. Normally such a protrusion is innocuous and the small piece of gut which has herniated can be gently reduced with no problem. However, unfortunately on occasions, the piece of gut may be lodged so firmly in the hernial sac outside the abdominal cavity as to be irreducible. Where

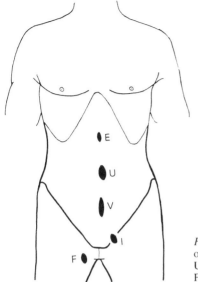

Figure 9.5 Common sites of occurrence of hernias: E = Epigastric; U = Umbilical; V = Ventral; I = Inguinal; F = Femoral.

a hernia is irreducible, two complications can occur, first, the passage of food through the portion of the intestine which is trapped may be obstructed and secondly the loop of the trapped intestine may be squeezed so tightly as to have its blood supply obstructed (a strangulated hernia). Under these latter circumstances unless the trapped hernia is released and its blood supply restored the incarcerated portion of gut becomes infarcted.

Treatment of hernias consists of the surgical repair of the weakened area in the wall of the abdominal cavity which means that the organ, e.g., the gut, can no longer herniate through. Usually when a patient has a hernia diagnosed he is put on a surgical waiting list, and subsequently admitted for an elective repair. However, some hernias are dealt with as emergencies, i.e., when they have become obstructed or strangulated, the patient usually being admitted with acute abdominal pain.

Malabsorption

Where the process of digestion and absorption of food is interfered with by a disease process such as Crohn's disease, the patient suffers weight loss, chronic abdominal pain and persistent diarrhoea. This condition is known as the malabsorption (i.e., poor absorption) syndrome and can be caused by many different disorders. Apart from Crohn's disease, such things as major surgery to the gut with the removal of large portions of that structure may cause it, as may diseases of the biliary tract and pancreas. The treatment of the condition consists of, where possible, curing the underlying disorder and in the meantime supplying the patient with the necessary nutrients which he is not absorbing from his gut in other ways, e.g., vitamin B_{12} by injection.

Crohn's disease

This is a chronic disorder of unknown causation which can affect any part of the gastrointestinal tract from beginning to end. It results in inflammation of the gut wall which therefore becomes thickened and sometimes also ulcerated. The patient's complaints are of feeling generally unwell with chronic recurrent abdominal pain, diarrhoea and sometimes the passage of blood per rectum. Complications occur not infrequently and include such things as obstruction or fistula formation. A fistula is an unnatural connection between two structures, most commonly it is between two different parts of the gut, e.g., the jejunum and colon, but it may be between the gut and other structures, e.g., large intestine and bladder, bladder and vagina, etc. Other complications of Crohn's disease include perforation, and gastrointestinal tract haemorrhage.

Treatment consists of administering a high fibre diet with associated vitamin and iron supplements to counteract the malabsorption. Where necessary, if the patient is seriously ill, he may be treated with steroids, (e.g., prednisolone/prednisone). The majority of patients with Crohn's end up having some form of surgery during the course of the disease mainly to treat the complications which occur, such as obstruction or perforation.

Ulcerative colitis

Like Crohn's disease this disorder is a chronic inflammatory disease of the gut of unknown causation which is confined to the colon and rectum. The patient usually presents with recurrent diarrhoea, the motion often having a high percentage of blood and mucus. Abdominal pain occurs and the patient often complains of feeling unwell with loss of weight and appetite. Complications of the disease include severe haemorrhage and perforation, however the most worrying problem is the fact that patients with the disease have a higher than normal incidence of carcinoma of the colon. Treatment of the disorder is with steroids and such drugs as sulphasalazine, though total removal of the colon (colectomy) is used in a significant number of cases.

Appendicitis

The appendix is a blind ended, worm-like structure about 10 cm, 4 inches long which comes off the caecum and lies in the right iliac fossa. Under certain circumstances, e.g., when the opening gets blocked, the appendix becomes inflamed and appendicitis is the result. A typical history is of a young person around 25 years of age, who may have had the odd attack of abdominal pain over the last week or so which was not severe, but who now has an acute attack which is often associated with some nausea and vomiting. The pain which was initially centrally placed in the abdomen becomes localized in the right iliac fossa and may become more severe. On examination the patient usually has a fever and a tachycardia, and when the abdomen is palpated, marked tenderness is noted in the right iliac fossa, the patient wincing and tensing his abdominal muscles (guarding) to prevent excessive pressure being applied over the painful region. In the uncomplicated case a plain abdominal X-ray has little to offer in the way of helpful information but if treatment is delayed the appendix may rupture and then gas from the bowel may be seen in the abdominal cavity localizing underneath the diaphragm, and the patient will develop a generalized peritonitis. If the patient's white cell count is checked it will usually show an increase in the number of cells present. Treatment is by emergency appendicectomy.

Haemorrhoids

These are very common, and are dilated veins in the region of the anal canal. They develop internally or externally and can cause pain, irritation and bleeding. Whilst various creams, ointments and suppositories may be used to ease the symptoms the condition can only be cured by injecting the veins or by their removal (haemorrhoidectomy).

Malignant disease of the gastrointestinal tract

The oesophagus

Here the developing tumour will start to block the lumen of the oesophagus and will result in the patient finding it difficult to swallow (dysphagia). At first it is only large lumps of food which will get stuck whilst things like milk puddings, soup and drinks pass through with no problem. Later, as the tumour increases in size less and less is able to pass through until at last even water is blocked. These tumours may also bleed and the patient may therefore present with a haematemesis. Diagnosis is made by performing a Barium Swallow, and then by oesophagoscopy. The only treatment is total removal of the tumour but this is rarely possible, the tumour having frequently ulcerated through the oesophagus to produce secondary tumours locally in the chest.

Carcinoma of the stomach

As the stomach is a large hollow organ, tumours can attain quite a significant size growing inwards into the cavity before they produce any symptoms. However if the tumour is sited at the exit to the stomach (the pylorus) it can rapidly produce obstruction. If it becomes ulcerated it may bleed and produce a haematemesis and/or melaena or if it spreads widely, producing secondary tumours throughout the abdominal cavity and in the liver, as is frequently the case, then the patient may present with loss of weight or appetite. This may be accompanied by chronic abdominal pain, and swelling of the abdomen, due to the presence of a large collection of fluid in the abdominal cavity (ascites). Diagnosis is by Barium Meal and gastroscopy, surgery is the only treatment and only about 2 per cent of patients survive 5 years.

Carcinoma of the colon and rectum

Tumours of the large intestine also have the potential to grow to quite a size before they produce symptoms. Common complaints are of alteration of bowel habit, (i.e., a patient who has normally had his bowels open daily for most of his life suddenly becomes constipated), bleeding per rectum and abdominal pain. Though diagnosis may be confirmed by Barium Enema or by endoscopy, a high percentage of tumours in the rectum may be palpated by an internal examination of that structure with a single finger. Treatment is surgical with removal of the diseased section of the gut and then either joining the severed ends together or closing up the rectal end and bringing the other end out through the anterior abdominal wall (a colostomy).

Chapter 10

Disorders of the liver, pancreas and spleen

Anatomy and physiology

These three organs all lie in the upper part of the abdominal cavity and are functionally inter-related (*see Figure 10.1*).

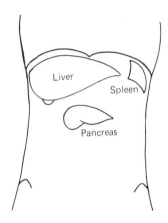

Figure 10.1 Diagram to illustrate relative positions of organs in the abdominal cavity.

The liver

This is the largest organ in the human body and has many functions including the production of some of the proteins found in the blood (e.g., albumin, fibrinogen, etc), the storage and release of sugars, the metabolism and the detoxification of many substances such as drugs, and the formation and excretion of bile, a greenish fluid produced by the breakdown of old blood cells.

The pancreas

This gland has two entirely separate functions, one is related to the production of the hormone insulin and is discussed in Chapter 13, the other is the production of enzymes to aid in the digestion of food as mentioned in Chapter 9. These enzymes are formed in the pancreas and secreted into the pancreatic duct which joins with the bile duct (*see Figure 10.2*) to form a common channel which opens into the duodenum.

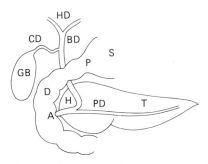

Figure 10.2 Diagrammatic representation of Bile and Pancreatic ducts: HD = Right and left hepatic ducts coming from the right and left lobes of the liver and joining to form: BD = The common bile duct; CD = The cystic duct to the gall-bladder; GB = Gall-bladder; D = Duodenum; A = The ampulla. The orifice through which bile and pancreatic juice enter the duodenum; P = Pylorus; S = Stomach; H = Head of the pancreas; T = Tail of the pancreas; PD = Pancreatic Duct.

Thus bile, manufactured in the liver, is stored in the gall-bladder until food reaches the first part of the duodenum. When this happens, bile is secreted from the gallbladder together with pancreatic juice from the pancreas and both are passed into the duodenum. There they blend with the food and aid in the splitting up of starches and fats into tiny pieces suitable for absorption into the blood stream from the gut.

The spleen

The spleen has a function in both the production and the destruction of red blood corpuscles and also in the formation of certain antibodies which are part of the body's defence mechanism. Unlike the liver or pancreas the spleen is not absolutely essential to life and people can survive even if it has to be removed due to injury.

Clinical features of diseases of the liver, pancreas and spleen

Abdominal pain is a common symptom of disease of the liver and its associated gallbladder, the pain being situated either in the right hypochondrium or in the epigastrium. Another wellknown feature of liver disease is jaundice, which occurs when a patient is not able to pass the bile produced by the liver into the gut. This is sometimes due to the blockage of the bile duct by a stone and results in the bile leaking into the blood stream and then out into the tissues of the body, which gives the patient a yellowish tinge. Jaundice is best detected in the sclera (whites of the eyes) which become light yellow in colour. The urine of a patient with jaundice is also full of bile and tends to be very dark in colour. Disease of the pancreas can also present with jaundice as for instance when a tumour grows in that organ and squeezes shut the duct carrying the flow of pancreatic juice and bile to the duodenum. The other common symptom of pancreatic disease is abdominal pain which may be acute, as in acute pancreatitis, or chronic.

Diseases which cut off the flow of bile and pancreatic juice to the gut also result in the occurrence of steatorrhea, where the motions are light in colour (due to the absence of bile) and much bulkier than usual as there is a large amount of undigested food (due to the absence of bile and pancreatic enzymes).

Disorders which affect the spleen alone are very rare but can cause pain and tenderness in the left hypochondrium.

Investigation of diseases of the liver, pancreas and spleen

Tests on urine and blood can indicate disease of the liver, for instance the presence of high levels of bilirubin (one of the constituents of bile) in either of these fluids. There are other blood tests of liver function and the liver may also be visualized using isotope, ultrasound, CAT or NMR scans as, with varying degrees of success, may the pancreas and spleen.

The gallbladder may be visualized by injecting the patient intravenously with a dye which concentrates itself in the biliary system, and X-rays taken subsequently outline the gallbladder and its associated ducts. This examination is known as a cholecystogram.

Another very useful investigation of liver function is to remove a small portion of the organ through a fine hollow needle (a liver biopsy), this piece of tissue may then be studied microscopically and biochemically.

When the pancreas is damaged, an enzyme, amylase, which is manufactured in the gland leaks out and high levels may be detected in the blood and urine.

Specific disorders

Hepatitis

This is a virus disease of the liver which is, generally speaking, mild and from which recovery is usually complete. The disorder begins with a fever and the patient feels generally unwell, lethargic and may appear to have an upset gastrointestinal system with nausea, vomiting and diarrhoea. Following this the patient's urine darkens in colour and he becomes jaundiced. Usually the disorder settles down over 3–4 weeks and in the uncomplicated case no active treatment is necessary. The disease may be caused by two types of virus, type A or type B, the latter is the more serious and can lead, in occasional cases, to a chronic infection. This type of hepatitis (type B) may be transmitted in minute quantities of blood and can occur after injections with unsterile needles (e.g., as occurs amongst drug addicts), or by the administration of blood which is contaminated by the virus.

The diagnosis of hepatitis will be confirmed by tests of liver function and by finding antibodies to hepatitis in the blood.

Cirrhosis

Cirrhosis of the liver can occur following damage to that organ by several different processes. For instance, after hepatitis (type B), over-indulgence in alcohol which is an hepatic poison, and after exposure to various drugs and chemicals which are also hepato-toxic, e.g., carbon tetrachloride. In this condition, instead of the organ being made up entirely of healthy active liver cells, there are many bands of tough fibrous tissue crisscrossing the structure with islands of functioning liver cells between them. The fibrosis occurs in areas of the liver which have been damaged by the disease process, and the patient with cirrhosis therefore has far fewer active liver cells than normal. Whilst these can carry out their tasks adequately for a while, the patient's liver function usually gradually deteriorates, particularly for instance if someone with alcoholic cirrhosis keeps drinking, and he goes into liver failure and dies. Diagnosis is confirmed by the finding of abnormal liver function tests combined with the characteristic picture on microscopic examination of the liver biopsy. There is at present no treatment which can reverse the damage to the liver caused by cirrhosis.

Cholecystitis

By cholecystitis we mean an inflammation of the gallbladder which usually occurs when the ducts leaving that structure become obstructed, often by a gallstone. Secondary to this obstruction the ducts become infected by bacteria which produce the inflammation. The patient usually presents with pain over the area of the gallbladder (i.e., just beneath the rib cage on the right), nausea or vomiting, and a fever, and is sometimes slightly jaundiced.

Plain X-ray films of the abdomen may demonstrate the gallstones and these may also be detected by ultrasound scans, or the diseased gallbladder visualized by a cholecystogram.

Treatment consists of giving analgesics for the pain, the eradication of any infection with antibiotics, and then when the condition has settled, consideration can be given to surgical removal of the gallbladder (cholecystectomy) if necessary.

Tumours

Whilst primary tumours of the liver do occur, it is much more common to find that malignant growths in the organ are secondary to tumours which have originated elsewhere. For instance, a carcinoma of the bronchus which originates in the lung, then spreads (metastasizes) to the liver. The liver is commonly involved when malignant tumours have disseminated widely as also are the lungs, these secondary tumours are known as metastases.

Pancreatitis

The main causes of this condition, which may be acute or chronic, are over indulgence in alcohol on a long term basis, or the presence of gallstones. In the acute attack the patient complains of severe abdominal pain of sudden onset, the pain being epigastric in situation, sometimes radiating through to the back, and accompanied by nausea and vomiting. The diagnosis is confirmed by finding raised levels of the enzyme amylase in the blood and/or urine, whilst a plain X-ray of the abdomen may demonstrate gallstones.

Chronic pancreatitis is a relapsing disorder with recurring bouts of abdominal pain often precipitated by a 'binge'.

There are often no specific treatments for either acute or chronic pancreatitis and therapy is merely supportive, e.g., analgesics for pain, replacement i.v. fluids, etc.

Carcinoma of the head of the pancreas

The pancreas is divided anatomically into a head and a tail. The head is intimately related to the combined pancreatic-bile duct, and when a malignancy arises in the gland, it is usually situated at this site. In view of the close proximity of the duct to the tumour, that structure is frequently slowly squeezed shut as the tumour enlarges, and as no bile can be excreted, the patient becomes jaundiced. The prognosis for this type of malignancy is very poor as complete removal of the tumour is rarely possible.

Disorders of the spleen

This structure is only rarely the primary site of disease, much more commonly it becomes enlarged, secondary to diseases in other systems such as cirrhosis of the liver, leukaemia, lymphoma, haemolytic anaemia, etc. However, the spleen can often be a problem where injuries to the left side of the abdomen and chest have occurred, as it may be ruptured and bleed profusely necessitating its urgent removal. Occasionally the rupture may be delayed and bleeding may not occur until 12 to 24 hours after the injury was sustained.

Chapter 11

The urinary system

Anatomy and physiology

The urinary system consists of:

(1) The kidneys which produce urine and which are supplied with blood by the renal artery. Blood leaves the kidney by the renal vein.
(2) The ureters which convey the urine from the kidney to the bladder.
(3) The bladder which acts as a reservoir.
(4) The urethra, for discharge of urine from the bladder (*see Figure 11.1*).

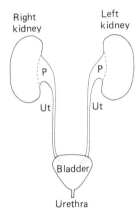

Right kidney   Left kidney

P   P

Ut   Ut

Bladder

Urethra

Figure 11.1 The urinary tract: Ut = Ureter; P = Pelvis of kidney.

Urine is a solution which contains some of the waste products produced by the normal body processes, e.g. urea. It also has amongst its constituents some of the elements and compounds found in normal body fluids, e.g., sodium, potassium, chloride, etc, which may be present in excess.

The kidneys lie on the posterior abdominal wall, mainly in the upper lumbar region, one on each side of the vertebral column deeply embedded in fat, behind the peritoneum. Each kidney measures 10–12 cm (4–5 inches) in length and 7 cm (2½ inches) in breadth, and in the adult weighs around 110–170 g (4–6 ounces). The kidney on the right is positioned slightly lower than that on the left and the inner side or hilum of the kidney is directed towards the vertebral column. Both blood vessels and the ureter enter and leave the kidney at the hilum (*see Figure 11.2*) whilst each kidney is surmounted by an adrenal (suprarenal) gland.

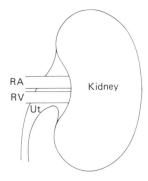

Figure 11.2 The Kidney: RA = Renal Artery; RV = Renal Vein; Ut = Ureter.

The kidneys are a dark reddish-brown in colour and consist of two regions, an outer cortex and an inner medulla. The kidney is made up of millions of glomeruli which are the functional units of the organ and which act as tiny filters. Blood enters the kidney via the renal artery and is filtered through the glomeruli, the waste products and excess substances being removed at this time. The urine so produced trickles down the ureters gradually filling the bladder which when full contracts and the urine is passed along the urethra to the exterior. This voiding process is known as micturition. The kidneys filter about 1 *l* (2 pints) of blood every minute and by varying the amount of chemicals that they remove they can adjust the chemical composition of the blood. Normally 1–2 *l* (2–4 pints) of urine a day is produced by an adult, however this volume will vary widely. It consists mainly of a solution of urea and sodium chloride, and in the absence of disease such abnormal constituents as protein and sugar would not be found.

Clinical features of urinary tract disease

One of the commonest symptoms associated with urinary tract disease is *frequency*, which is the repeated passage of urine with only short intervals between each micturition. Frequency is often accompanied by dysuria, or pain on micturition. The pain of dysuria is usually described as being burning or stinging. Another clinical feature of urinary tract disease associated with dysuria is haematuria or the passage of blood in the urine.

Pain and tenderness in the area overlying the site of the kidneys (loin pain) is seen in pyelonephritis and this may be confused with the pain of renal colic. In renal colic the patient experiences very severe pain of acute onset which is initially felt in the loin and which radiates down into the groin.

Polyuria, the passage of large quantities of urine, occurs occasionally, as does oliguria which is the production and passage of small quantities of urine (i.e., less than 500 ml (1 pint) in 24 hours). This is a serious sign in urinary tract disease as obviously is anuria, when no urine at all is produced.

A condition which is sometimes confused with anuria is retention of urine. Under these circumstances urine is produced by the kidneys and arrives in the bladder but is unable to leave that structure usually due to compression of the urethra by an enlarged prostate gland.

Investigation of urinary tract disease

Kidney function may be tested by measuring the amount of urine produced by the patient, and also by estimating the concentration of the waste products which are excreted. Normal urine tested using specially impregnated paper strips will be found not to contain any of the proteins normally found in the blood. However, in the presence of infection of the urinary tract, and also where there has been structural damage to the kidney by some disease process, e.g., glomerulonephritis, the urine may be found to be heavily loaded with proteins. When an infection is suspected it will be worthwhile attempting to grow the bacteria thought to be causing the infection from a fresh sample of urine.

Blood tests are used to estimate the level of such things as urea, sodium etc., and abnormalities may reveal a malfunction of the kidney.

Whilst a plain X-ray of the abdomen may reveal a stone causing renal colic, if it is wished to visualize the kidneys themselves the patient has to be given an intravenous injection of a radio-opaque dye which concentrates in the kidney and is excreted by it. This investigation is known as an intravenous pyelogram (IVP). The kidneys and bladder may also be visualized by isotope, ultrasound and CAT scans.

The kidney may of course also be biopsied by inserting a hollow needle into the organ and removing a small piece of tissue for examination under the microscope. The needle is pushed in through the loin over the site of the kidney.

Specific renal disorders

Urinary tract infections

These are very common problems, more so amongst women than men, and may be manifested as pyelonephritis where the seat of the infection is in the kidney or cystitis where the seat of the infection is in the bladder. Pyelonephritis is much the more serious infection, the patient feels unwell, is feverish and sometimes has acute shivering attacks (rigors). There is pain in the loin associated with tenderness in that area and there may be symptoms of cystitis (see below) as well. Pyelonephritis may be acute or chronic, the acute attack will be more dramatic but in fact may be occurring on top of a smouldering chronic infection which has persisted and is gradually destroying the kidney.

Cystitis is a frequently occurring disorder particularly amongst women and is characterized by the frequent urge to pass urine. Only small quantities of urine are passed at any one time and its passage is very painful (dysuria), the patient describing it as burning or stinging. Such individuals are not usually systematically ill but a bout of cystitis can be very debilitating due to the pain.

The diagnosis of a UTI is confirmed by examining the urine and finding it looking cloudy as it is loaded with white blood cells released into the urine from the blood stream in order to fight the infection. Protein will be found on testing the urine (proteinuria) and the infecting organism may be grown in the Bacteriology Laboratory. Treatment is then by the use of the appropriate antibiotic, e.g., cotrimoxazole (Septrin), amoxycillin (Amoxil), etc. to which the organism is sensitive.

Renal calculi (stones)

Kidney stones form in the urine as it lies in the pelvis of the kidney. The stones are initially just tiny crystals which unless passed to the exterior at this stage can grow very quickly to become the size of small pieces of gravel. If they then begin to travel down the ureter, that structure is stretched and scraped and this results in the pain known as renal colic. Renal colic starts in the loin and radiates down into the groin. The pain is very severe and tends to wax and wane, often being associated with haematuria. The diagnosis can frequently be confirmed by taking a plain X-ray of the abdomen and observing the small radio-opaque stone lying somewhere along the line of passage of the ureter.

Treatment consists of relieving the patient's pain with a strong analgesic, e.g. pethidine, and making sure that plenty of fluids are consumed, which will encourage the stone to pass into the bladder. Usually under these circumstances the stone is passed via the urethra, however, if it does not appear, surgical intervention may be necessary.

Glomerulonephritis

In this condition there is an inflammatory reaction in the glomeruli of the kidney and white blood cells are released from the blood stream to infiltrate the area. The precise reason for the occurrence of this inflammation is unknown but it does not appear to be due to an infection with bacteria or viruses. The main problem associated with this disorder is that the damage caused to the kidney over a period of years leads to chronic renal failure. Glomerulonephritis may be present for some time before it presents with gradually worsening oedema, or it may be discovered when an otherwise symptomless patient is found to have protein in his urine on a routine examination, e.g., for insurance purposes. Sometimes presentation is more acute with gross oedema and/or haematuria, the oedema often being particularly marked in children who are afflicted with the disorder.

Diagnosis is confirmed by the finding of protein and/or blood in the urine and often, unfortunately, by evidence of renal failure being detected in blood samples. Precise diagnosis as to the type and severity of the disorder can only be made by renal biopsy which is essential in order to be able to give some sort of prognosis to the patient.

Renal failure

Renal failure may be acute or chronic.

Acute renal failure

By definition this condition comes on suddenly, usually secondary to some catastrophic event such as major blood loss from for instance an accidentally severed blood vessel, or perhaps a massive haemorrhage following child birth. This haemorrhage means that the supply of blood and hence of oxygen to the kidneys is necessarily reduced and the ischaemic kidney ceases to function. There are many other causes of acute renal failure including septicaemia (i.e., where bacteria have got into the blood stream and are multiplying) and drug toxicity as certain drugs have a damaging effect on the kidney (e.g., Amphoteracin B.)

The diagnosis is made by measuring the amount of urine produced and examining it biochemically and microscopically, and also checking the patient's blood for rising levels of urea together with abnormalities in the levels of such elements as potassium and sodium. IVPs are also often required as is renal biopsy.

The immediate treatment of renal failure consists of tackling the underlying cause, e.g., blood transfusion for haemorrhage, antibiotics for septicaemia. The definitive treatment for the kidney failure is renal dialysis. There are two types of dialysis, haemodialysis and peritoneal dialysis. In the former a small tube (a shunt) is inserted into an artery, such as the radial artery at the wrist, and blood led out of that into an artificial kidney machine. In the machine impurities are removed as well as excess body chemicals, such as potassium. The blood is then returned to the body via another tube inserted into a small vein in the same wrist. This is the best form of dialysis. Peritoneal dialysis is a rather cruder method and consists of inserting several litres of fluid into the peritoneal cavity. This fluid is left in the cavity for a few hours and leeches some of the impurities out from the blood prior to being drained out again. A special button is inserted in the anterior abdominal wall to facilitate this procedure. Both haemodialysis and peritoneal dialysis will of course have to be repeated frequently until the kidneys recover and start functioning properly again.

Chronic renal failure

As with acute renal failure this may have many causes, e.g., glomerulonephritis, chronic pyelonephritis, etc. It presents insidiously on top of the underlying disorder which has caused it. When the diagnosis has been confirmed, a decision has to be taken on which line of treatment to follow. Where possible the underlying condition, e.g., chronic pyelonephritis, is treated to prevent the deterioration of the minimal amount of function remaining, and then the patient's diet is adjusted to keep to a minimum the amount of toxic waste products produced. The critical decision is whether or not to enter the patient on a programme of chronic haemodialysis and/or renal transplantation. This decision can be a difficult one as the regime for treatment is complicated and facilities only located at a few specialist centres.

Prostatic hypertrophy

In men, after the urethra leaves the bladder, on its way to the exterior it passes through the prostate gland (*see Figure 11.3*). This

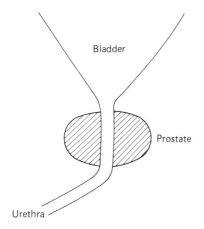

Figure 11.3 Diagrammatic representation of outflow tract from bladder.

gland which is part of the reproductive system sometimes increases in size in the elderly and compresses the urethra which is running through it. This increase in size may be due to simple hypertrophy (enlargement) or, less often, from a malignant tumour arising in the gland (carcinoma of the prostate) (*see Figure 11.4*). The consequent

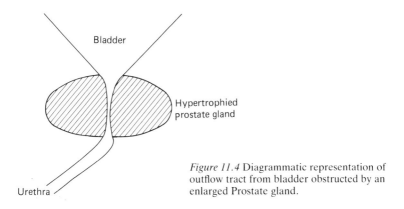

Figure 11.4 Diagrammatic representation of outflow tract from bladder obstructed by an enlarged Prostate gland.

narrowing of the urethra results in a difficulty in passing urine which only dribbles out slowly over several minutes. Only a small percentage of the bladder contents are passed at each attempt at micturition and this means that the patient makes frequent visits to the lavatory, spending a much longer time than usual on each visit. The treatment of the disorder consists of the partial or complete removal of the gland surgically.

Chapter 12

The musculoskeletal system

Anatomy

The two components of this system are so interlinked that they must be considered together. The skeleton consists of a large number of bones which are held together by tough fibrous ligaments, and where two bones meet a joint is formed. Bone is basically made up of a fibrous substance which is subsequently hardened by the deposition around it of crystals of salts such as calcium phosphate. Bone is not inert but is constantly being remodelled, old bone being absorbed and new bone laid down.

The bones which make up the skeleton serve four purposes:

(1) They form a stout solid framework upon which the shape of the body can be built up by the muscles.
(2) They are the rigid levers to which muscles are attached, and these muscles make movement possible by shortening and lengthening.
(3) They form bony cavities which protect vital organs, e.g. the intrathoracic cavity inside the ribs which protects the heart and lungs.
(4) The marrow in the central part of certain bones produces blood cells.

The skeleton is divided into two parts, the axial skeleton and the appendicular skeleton.

Axial skeleton

This consists of the skull, vertebral column and rib cage.

The skull

The skull (*see Figure 12.1*) is made up of several bones which are joined solidly together at immovable suture lines. At birth these bones are not yet fully grown and have not locked together. Under these circumstances there are 'soft' spots on the top of the skull which will be palpable in babies but which will disappear when the bones grow large enough to meet. These spaces are known as fontanelles and they close by around the age of 18 months.

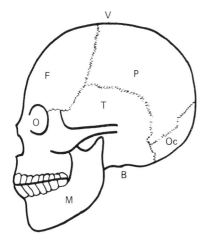

Figure 12.1 The skull: O = Orbit; F =
Frontal bone; P = Parietal bone; T =
Temporal bone; Oc = Occipital bone; M
= Mandible; V = Vertex (Top of the vault
of the skull); B = Base.

The skull is made up of three separate areas:

(1) The vault or top of the skull.
(2) The base which articulates (joins) with the vertebral column.
(3) The facial bones and mandible.

The vertebral column

The vertebral column is split up into five different areas. These are,
from the base of the skull down, first the cervical area (made up of
seven bones), then the thoracic or dorsal area (twelve bones) (*see
Figure 12.2*), thirdly the lumbar area (five bones), fourthly the
sacral area (five bones) and finally the coccygeal area (four bones).
The vertebrae of the first three areas are separated one from
another by the intervertebral discs (*see Figure 12.3*). These are
made of a tough springy material and form buffers between the
bones. The bones of the sacrum and coccyx have no such discs and
are fused (joined together) so that whilst theoretically they are
made up of nine separate bones, they are effectively just one solid
bony mass. The vertebrae enclose a central canal in their bony
framework and it is down this so-called spinal canal (*see Figure 12.4*)
that the extension of the brain, the spinal cord runs, giving off its
sensory and motor peripheral nerves.

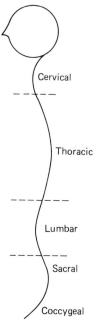

Cervical

Thoracic

Lumbar

Sacral

Coccygeal   *Figure 12.2* The regions of the spine

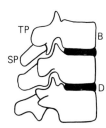

Figure 12.3 Three of the lumbar vertebrae from the side:
TP = Transverse process; SP = Spinous process; B = Body
of the vertebra; D = Intervertebral disc.

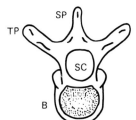

Figure 12.4 A single vertebra from above: TP =
Transverse process; SP = Spinous process; B = Body
of the vertebra; SC = Spinal canal (Down which the
spinal cord runs).

The thorax

The 12 ribs arise one from each of the thoracic (dorsal) vertebrae and run in a semi-circle to meet at the sternum (*see Figure 12.5*)

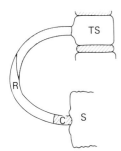

Figure 12.5 A single rib from the front: TS = Thoracic spine; S = Sternum; R = Rib; C = Costal cartilage.

forming a barrel-shaped structure (the thorax) which will enclose the heart and lungs (*see Figure 12.6*).

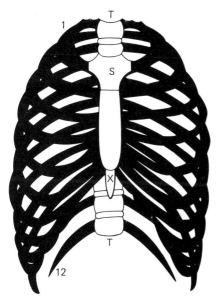

Figure 12.6 The thorax: T = Thoracic spine; S = Sternum; X = Xiphoid; 1 = First rib; 12 = Twelfth rib.

Appendicular skeleton

This is made up of two girdles (shoulder and pelvic) and the bones of the limbs. The shoulder girdle is made up of a broad flat scapula or shoulder blade and a short clavicle or collar bone. The clavicle articulates with the top of the sternum forming the sterno-clavicular joint and with part of the scapula known as the acromion, to form the acromio-clavicular joint which forms the upper surface of the shoulder (*see Figure 12.7*).

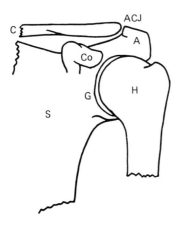

Figure 12.7 The shoulder joint: A = Acromion; Co = Coracoid and G = Glenoid (all parts of the scapula); S = Scapula; C = Clavicle; ACJ = Acromio-Clavicular joint; H = Humerus.

The shoulder joint itself is formed by articulation between the humerus, the bone of the upper arm, and a part of the scapula known as the glenoid fossa. The humerus, as well as having the shoulder joint at its upper end has the elbow joint at its lower end. This joint is formed between the humerus and the two bones of the forearm, the radius and ulna, which lie parallel to one another (*see Figure 12.8*).

At the lower end of the radius and ulna lies the wrist joint which is formed by the articulation of these two bones with the eight small bones which make up the carpus or wrist. The carpus also articulates with the metacarpals, the bones which form the palm of the hand. Finally we have the phalanges or finger bones, small bones of which there are three in each finger with two in the thumb (*see Figure 12.9*).

The pelvic girdle is formed from three bones, the ilium, ischium and pubis, on each side. These bones are fused together and at the back, this bony mass articulates with the sacrum to form the sacro-iliac joints and in front, the two halves of the pelvis meet at the symphysis pubis (*see Figure 12.10*). Articulating with the acetabulum of

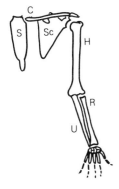

Figure 12.8 The shoulder girdle and arm: S = Sternum; Sc = Scapula; C = Clavicle; H = Humerus; R = Radius; U = Ulna.

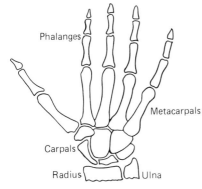

Figure 12.9 The hand

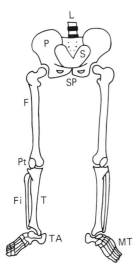

Figure 12.10 The pelvic girdle and lower limb: P = Pelvis; L = Lumbar spine; S = Sacrum; SP = Symphisis Pubis; F = Femur; Pt = Patella; T = Tibia; Fi = Fibula; Ta = Tarsus; Mt = Metatarsals.

the pelvis to form the hip joint is the femur or thigh bone, the largest bone in the body. Like the humerus it forms a joint at both ends and at its lower end lies the knee joint made with the two bones of the lower part of the leg, the tibia (or shin bone) and fibula. Protecting the knee joint from the front is the knee cap or patella. The tibia and fibula form the ankle at their lower end with the seven bones of the ankle or tarsus. The tarsus is equivalent to the carpus of the wrist, and the tarsus articulates with the five metatarsal bones which form the sole of the foot. The small bones which make up the toes have the same name as those which make up the fingers and are known as phalanges.

Joints

A joint is formed wherever two bones meet, however here we are only concerned with joints where movement is possible and not, for instance, with the joints formed where two of the bones of the skull meet. For a joint to function properly the following five features must be present as well as the two bones involved:

(1) The ends of the two bones which are going to rub together as the joints move, must be covered with a tough smooth substance to allow movement to take place with the minimum of friction so that the bones do not wear out. This substance is known as cartilage.

(2) The whole joint must be enclosed in a joint capsule lined by a membrane capable of secreting a lubricant (the synovial membrane).

(3) The joint space must be full of an oily lubricating fluid, synovial fluid, secreted by the synovial membrane.

(4) The bones which make up the joint must be firmly held together by ligaments, which sometimes form part of the joint capsule.

(5) Muscles must pass across the joint and these will, by alternately contracting (shortening) and relaxing (lengthening) move the limb.

There are two major types of joint to be considered: first, hinge joints and secondly ball and socket joints (*see Figure 12.11*). Hinge joints, e.g., knee joints and finger joints are somewhat limited in that they only permit the movements of flexion and extension whereas ball and socket joints, e.g. at the junction of femur and pelvis allow not only these movements but rotation as well, thus movement is possible in all planes at a ball and socket joint.

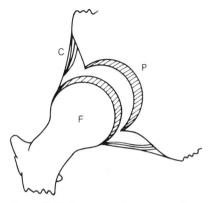

Figure 12.11 Diagrammatic representation
of a typical ball and socket joint. (The hip
joint): P = Pelvis; F = Femur; C = Ligaments
surrounding joint capsule. The ends of the
bones which form the joint are covered in
cartilage (cross-hatched), and the space
within the joint is full of a lubricant
(synovial fluid).

Muscles

There are three different types of muscle:

(1) Skeletal (striped) muscle is the type which makes up the bulk of
the body's muscle, and is the 'meat' on our bones. It is under
our direct control via the brain, spinal cord and peripheral
motor nerves.
(2) Smooth (unstriped) muscle is the type of muscle found in such
structures as the gut and bronchi, and which can for instance, by
contracting behind a lump of food, force it along the intestine.
This type of muscle is not under our direct control but is
regulated by the autonomic nervous system.
(3) Myocardium (heart) muscle is only found in the heart, and
again is under the control of the autonomic nervous system.

We shall in this chapter be confining ourselves to discussion of the
first of these three types of muscle.
Muscles are the structures, which by their ability to initially contract (shorten) and then relax (lengthen) cause joints to move. A
muscle will originate from the bone on one side of the joint and be
inserted into the bone on the other side of the joint and they tend to
be arranged in opposing groups. One group shortens to cause

flexion (the flexor muscles, e.g., biceps) while the opposing group lengthens to allow this movement (the extensor muscles, e.g., the triceps). Subsequently the movement is reversed and extension occurs by the shortening of the extensor muscles whilst the flexor muscles relax, lengthen, and allow the limb to return to its fully extended position. The muscle consists of a bulky 'belly' composed of muscle fibres and this then narrows down at its insertion to a tough tendon which is attached firmly to the bone.

Typical groups of muscles are the biceps which is situated on the front of the humerus and which flexes the elbow, and its opposing group of extensor muscles, the triceps, which lies on the back of the humerus and extends the elbow. In the leg, the quadriceps muscles, which make up the front of the thigh, extend the knee, and the hamstring muscles, which make up the back of the thigh, flex the knee.

Clinical features of diseases of the musculoskeletal system

The most commonly observed clinical features of disorders of bone are bone pain and joint pain which can be severe and intractable. Where joints are affected they may be swollen, distorted and stiff, often with gross restriction of their range of movement. Muscle disease is often manifested by weakness which may be associated with wasting of the muscles though occasionally the muscles may be swollen and tender.

Investigation of disease of the musculoskeletal system

The most useful investigation in diseases of the bones and joints are X-rays, but other types of radiological investigation such as isotope scans are sometimes useful. Some blood tests such as those which measure the levels of calcium and phosphate are also used.

Muscle disease is often confirmed by finding high levels of such enzymes as creatine kinese in the blood. High levels occur because these enzymes, which are normally confined within the muscle cells themselves, leak out into the blood stream when the cells are damaged by disease and thus may be detected there (cf myocardial infarction where enzymes leak out of damaged heart muscle). Another useful test of muscle function is to measure the electrical discharge produced when it functions, this test is known as an electromyogram (EMG) and is often accompanied by a muscle biopsy.

Specific disorders of the musculoskeletal system

The commonest problem associated with bones is a fracture, and this is dealt with in Chapter 16.

Arthritis

This implies disease of the joints and there are two major types of arthritis:

Osteoarthritis (OA)

In this condition, the cartilage which covers the ends of the bones which make up a joint becomes worn faster than it can be replaced and therefore the bones themselves rub together when the joint moves and this causes pain and inflammation (*see Figure 12.12*).

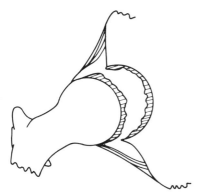

Figure 12.12 Osteo-arthritis in a ball and socket joint. The cartilage covering the bones is roughened and has been partly worn away (cf *Figure 12.11*).

The joints become swollen, stiff, painful and often, when the disorder affects the hands or limbs, they become deformed. Joints which are commonly affected are those of the hand, spine (particularly the cervical and lumbar regions) as well as the knees and hips. The diagnosis is usually confirmed by an X-ray of the affected joint.

The pain and stiffness of osteoarthritis is treated by any one of a number of anti-inflammatory drugs, e.g., ibuprofen (Brufen) diclofenac (Voltarol), etc. However, sometimes certain of the joints are so badly affected by wear and tear that artificial joints (prostheses), e.g., hips, knees, etc, have to be implanted surgically.

Rheumatoid arthritis (RA)

In this condition there is damage to the synovial membrane of the joints by the patient's own immune system. Normally the immune system forms antibodies which attack any micro-organisms, e.g., bacteria and viruses which invade the body. However, under certain unusual circumstances it can produce antibodies against the patient's own tissues, giving rise to what is known as an autoimmune disease.

In RA the joints commonly affected are those of the hands, wrists and knees, and as well as having morning stiffness and pain, the joints are frequently badly damaged by the disease and become markedly deformed.

Diagnosis is confirmed by the finding of an autoantibody in the blood and characteristic changes on X-ray.

Treatment is by the use of anti-inflammatory drugs as for OA and sometimes also, in severe cases corticosteroid drugs such as prednisolone may be used. When joints become badly damaged surgical replacement is sometimes carried out.

Osteomyelitis

This is caused by a bacterial infection in the bone and is always a serious matter as it is difficult to get antibiotics into the bone in high enough concentrations to kill the bacteria. The disease may result when bacteria, from for instance a boil in the skin, get into the blood stream and then settle in a bone elsewhere in the body. Alternatively, if a patient has a compound fracture and the exposed bone gets contaminated, infection frequently sets in and osteomyelitis results. If the acute osteomyelitis is not cleared up rapidly, by treatment with the appropriate antibiotic, it may become chronic and this condition can last for years defying prolonged antibiotic treatment and surgery. The infecting organism may be one of a wide variety of bacteria including that which causes tuberculosis. Where the infection involves a joint it is known as a septic arthritis.

Osteoporosis

In this common disorder bone becomes thin and therefore not as strong as it should be, the disorder being frequently found in post-menopausal women and because the bones are weaker than normal, fractures occur very easily (pathological fractures). The cause of this disorder is unknown and no really satisfactory treatment is at present available.

Paget's disease

Paget's disease is relatively common, however, as it is often symptomless, the patient is unaware that he has the disorder. In Paget's disease the bone becomes thicker and heavier, but, paradoxically, it is often less hard and this results for instance in a weight-bearing bone like the tibia bending (bowing) under the strain, giving the patient bow-legs. Most patients with this disorder do not require any treatment.

Bone tumours

Whilst primary bone tumours do occur they are less common than tumours which are secondary (metastases) having spread from primary malignancies most commonly of the lung, breast or prostate.

Diseases of muscle

Disorders which purely affect muscle are rare and consist mainly of various types of muscular dystrophy which result in gross weakness. Muscle may be affected secondarily by a disease such as polio which primarily affects the nerves. Under these circumstances the nerve which is damaged does not any longer conduct motor impulses to the muscle it innervates and this consequently does not move, so that the muscle atrophies (wastes). Similar disuse atrophy occurs in a limb which is put into a plaster cast for a month or two to allow fractured bones to heal.

Chapter 13

The endocrine system

Anatomy and physiology

The endocrine system consists of a group of six glands all of which differ in structure and function, and which are situated in different parts of the body (*see Figure 13.1*). These glands have one thing in common however, and this is that they produce one or more *hormones*. A hormone is a chemical messenger which is produced in a gland, e.g., the parathyroids, then released into the blood stream to produce its effect on another organ or tissue somewhere else in the body. In the case of the parathyroid hormone this target tissue is bone.

The most important gland is the pituitary as it acts as a 'master gland' producing several hormones each of which has a role to play in the production of hormones in another gland, e.g., thyroid stimulating hormone (TSH) is produced in the pituitary and acts on the thyroid, stimulating it in turn to produce its own hormone thyroxine.

The pituitary

This gland is sited in the base of the brain and may be considered to be made up of two parts, the anterior and the posterior pituitary.

Anterior pituitary

This part of the gland produces the following hormones:

(1) Adrenocorticotrophic hormone (ACTH). The targets for this hormone are the adrenal glands which are stimulated to produce corticosteroids.
(2) Thyroid stimulating hormone (TSH). This hormone is aimed at the thyroid gland stimulating it to produce thyroxine.
(3) Gonadotrophines. These are targeted on the gonads (ovaries

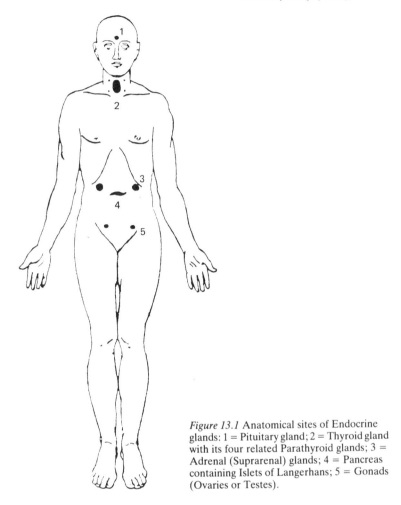

Figure 13.1 Anatomical sites of Endocrine glands: 1 = Pituitary gland; 2 = Thyroid gland with its four related Parathyroid glands; 3 = Adrenal (Suprarenal) glands; 4 = Pancreas containing Islets of Langerhans; 5 = Gonads (Ovaries or Testes).

and testes) which they stimulate into producing germ cells (ova and spermatazoa).

(4) Growth hormone. The function of this hormone is obvious, under-production in childhood leads to dwarfism.

Posterior pituitary

This structure is the site of release of two hormones:
(1) Anti-diuretic (ADH). The target organ for this hormone is the kidney where it acts to minimize the amount of water lost.

(2) Oxytocin which is a hormone that causes the pregnant uterus to contract thus initiating labour.

Other glands

The thyroid

This produces thyroxine, a hormone which stimulates the metabolism of the body as a whole and which has a role in ensuring normal growth and development. Thyroxine has iodine built into its structure and for the proper functioning of the thyroid gland the patient must receive an adequate dietary intake of iodine. If this is not present, hypofunction of the gland results, with consequent enlargement of that structure, the so called goitre.

The parathyroids

There are four of these glands which produce the substance known as parathormone. This hormone controls the level of calcium in the body and hence is linked to bone metabolism. It is not controlled by the pituitary.

The gonads (ovaries and testes)

These produce the hormones oestrogen and progesterone in the female and testosterone in the male. The hormones are essential for normal sexual development and function.

The adrenal glands

Like the pituitary the adrenals are also divided into two parts: (see Figure 13.2)

(1) The cortex or outer part which produces two types of hormones:
    (a) Aldosterone which is used to control the level of sodium in the blood.
    (b) Cortisol which is used to control the metabolism of proteins, carbohydrates and fats and is particularly important at times of stress. It also reduces inflammation and allergic responses.
(2) The medulla or central part (see Figure 13.2) which produces the catecholamines, adrenaline and noradrenaline, substances which activate the sympathetic nervous system causing an increase in heart rate, blood pressure, etc.

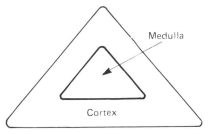

Figure 13.2 Diagrammatic representation of a
section through the Adrenal.

The pancreas

The bulk of this organ is concerned with the production of enzymes used in the digestion of food. Scattered throughout the gland however are small groups of cells, the islets of Langerhans which produce the hormone insulin. This substance controls the level of sugar in the blood.

Clinical features of endocrine disorders

With such a wide variety of functions being controlled by these organs, the signs and symptoms of endocrine disorders are many and varied, however the following list covers the major clinical features:

(1) Rapid weight loss. This can occur in diabetes and hyper-thyroidism.
(2) Obesity. This is a feature of Cushing's Syndrome.
(3) Tiredness of recent origin which is a feature of hypoethyroidism and adrenal insufficiency amongst other things.
(4) Delayed growth/sexual development may well have an endocrine cause.

Investigation of endocrine disease

The major investigations for endocrine disorders are the estimation of the levels of the various hormones in the blood and/or urine, e.g., the level of thyroxine in the blood or the level of adrenocortico-steroids in the urine. Sometimes the estimation may be an indirect one, e.g., measuring the level of the sugar in the blood can give us some idea as to whether or not insulin is being produced by the pancreas.

Specific endocrine disorders

There are essentially two types of disorder, one where the organ is secreting too much of the hormone it manufactures, this is known as hyperfunction, e.g., hyperthyroidism. The other is where the gland is not secreting enough of the hormone, this being known as hypofunction, e.g., hypothyroidism.

Hypopituitarism

This may arise from one of two causes. First, a tumour or cyst may develop and enlarge in the region of the pituitary gland, gradually crushing it, or alternatively, the gland may become infarcted in a patient who is shocked. The onset of signs and symptoms is insidious, women cease menstruating and men become impotent, body hair disappears and men have to shave much less frequently. Next the signs and symptoms of thyroid failure (page 123) appear and finally those of adrenal failure (page 124).

The diagnosis is made by detecting a cyst or tumour in the pituitary region on a skull X-ray or a scan, and this is accompanied by low levels of various hormones in the blood stream.

Treatment consists of, where possible, removing the cyst or tumour, or destroying it by radiation therapy. This is then followed by replacement of the missing thyroid, adrenal and sex hormones.

Hyperpituitarism

This is again usually due to a tumour which develops in the pituitary and which over-secretes a particular hormone. This can manifest itself in a variety of ways depending upon which hormone is being produced in excess.

Excess growth hormone (GH)

If this occurs in a child where the growing points of the bones are still active, gigantism results, the patient becoming tall and powerfully built. Where the growth hormone is overproduced in an adult in whom the growing points of the bones have closed, the patient's height does not increase but there is an overgrowth of bone and other organs and tissues, such as the liver, tongue, lips, etc. This disorder is known as Acromegaly and it leads to characteristic facial appearance.

Excess adrenocorticotrophin (ACTH)

This leads to an excessive secretion of adrenocorticosteroids from the adrenal gland and results in Cushing's Syndrome (page 124).

Treatment consists of the removal of the tumour or its destruction by radiation. Hormone replacement therapy is then indicated as the patient will have hypopituitarism, the pituitary gland having been destroyed. Unfortunately however, the physical appearances produced in acromegaly and gigantism cannot be reversed.

Hypothyroidism

An insufficiency of thyroid hormone in the newborn results in the disorder known as cretinism, if the problem is not detected early the child will be both physically and mentally retarded. If the insufficiency only develops in adult life, the condition is known as myxoedema. This is more common in women and the patient becomes lethargic (physically and intellectually), the voice becomes gruff and the face rather pale and puffy. The patient, who is usually elderly, feels the cold easily and may become hypothermic in wintery weather.

The diagnosis is made by the measurement of the amount of hormone (thyroxine) present in the blood and treatment is straight forward, being simple replacement of the deficient hormone in tablet form.

Hyperthyroidism

This results where there is an over secretion of thyroid hormone, and the most striking physical sign is the 'pop-eyed' expression that many patients with the disorder have. The problem occurs much more commonly amongst women than men and comes on gradually. The patient is easily agitated, feels warm even in circumstances where 'normal' people feel cool, and often has a rapid pulse which is sometimes irregular due to the presence of atrial fibrillation.

Diagnosis is based on the estimation of the amount of circulating thyroxine in the blood and treatment is via one of three ways. First, surgical with partial removal of the gland, secondly by giving the patient tablets which damp down the activity of the gland and thirdly by administering small doses of radioactive iodine which is taken up by the thyroid and destroys some of the gland without the necessity of surgery.

Hypoparathyroidism

This occurs very rarely, usually as a result of damage to the glands at the time of surgery on the thyroid. It results in too low a level of calcium in the blood.

Hyperparathyroidism

This usually occurs due to a small benign tumour growing in one of the parathyroid glands and results in the amount of calcium circulating in the blood being raised. This calcium is removed from bones making them softer than normal and more likely to fracture. Another feature of the disorder is renal colic, as the high level of calcium causes small renal stones to develop in the kidney (page 102). Diagnosis is made by measuring the level of calcium and phosphate in the blood and also that of parathormone. Treatment is by removal of the enlarged gland.

Hypoadrenalism (Addison's Disease)

This is due to the destruction of the adrenals by one of several disease processes, and is a rare condition. The patient, usually female, presents with vague complaints of weakness and lethargy, sometimes accompanied by abnormal skin pigmentation. Diagnosis is made by measuring the amount of cortisol in the blood before and after an injection of synthetic ACTH, and treatment is by replacement of the missing hormones.

Hyperadrenalism (Cushing's Syndrome)

This disorder results from an oversecretion of cortisol from the adrenal cortex. This may occur due to the overproduction of ACTH from a pituitary tumour which stimulates overproduction of cortisol from the adrenals, or via a tumour developing in the adrenal cortex itself. Cushing's Syndrome also occurs when a patient is prescribed synthetic hormones, e.g., prednisolone for a disorder such as Rheumatoid Arthritis or asthma. If the patient has to be on a high dose for an extended period the characteristic appearance of the disorder, obesity, a round 'moon' face, ankle swelling, excessive hair growth, weakness and bruising, will develop. Diagnosis is made by confirming the excessive production of cortisol and treatment consists of removal of the tumour where possible. Where the appearances are due to steroid treatment, attempts are made to reduce the dose of prednisolone to the minimum possible which will control the underlying disease, e.g., asthma.

Phaeochromocytoma

Very rarely a tumour appears in the adrenal medulla, and this produces an excess of the catecholamines, adrenaline and noradrenaline. These tumours give rise to episodes of hypertension and cardiac arrhythmias and they can be diagnosed by measuring the levels of the hormones in the blood and/or urine. Treatment is surgical removal.

Disorders of the gonadal function

These occur sometimes due to faulty hormone secretion or balance, they are not life threatening but can cause great distress when they produce infertility.

Diabetes mellitus

When a carbohydrate-containing food, such as bread, is eaten, it is broken down in the stomach and small intestine into sugars by the action of chewing in the mouth, churning in the stomach and by the enzymes in the secretions produced by these structures. The sugars are absorbed into the blood stream from the small intestine and thus the level of sugar in the blood rises. This rise in the level of the blood-sugar is detected as the blood passes through the islets of Langerhans in the pancreas, as they are constantly sampling the blood which passes through them. When the islets detect a rise in blood-sugar levels they begin to secrete the hormone insulin into the blood.

Sugar is a vital ingredient for the production of energy in all the cells of the various organs and tissues in the body. The sugar is transported throughout the body by the blood stream and insulin is the substance which helps take the sugar out of the blood and put it into the cells of the body for use in producing energy. Thus when the islets put insulin into the blood it helps the cells to take in the sugar they need and consequently the level of sugar in the blood drops slowly back to lie around its normal base level.

Diabetes mellitus occurs when the islets of Langerhans in the pancreas are not producing enough insulin. Under these circumstances the levels of sugar in the blood remains higher than normal, and the cells cannot obtain the sugar they need in sufficient quantities for energy production.

Diabetic patients may be divided into two groups, those who present as young people and who are generally thin and who have the type of diabetes mellitus which can be difficult to control. The second group are those whose diabetes does not come on until late middle-age and who have a milder form of the disorder, they tend to be overweight and their disease is much easier to control.

The disease in young people often presents with a history of fairly rapid weight loss accompanied by polyuria (passing large quantities of urine), and polydipsia (drinking a great deal). The diagnosis is made by finding sugar in the urine and a persistently raised level of sugar in the blood.

Treatment of diabetes mellitus can be in one of three ways depending upon the severity of the disease. Mild diabetes may be controlled by the use of a suitable diet which can be tailored to the individual patient. Where the diabetic is overweight, his diet may be weight-reducing and the patient may find that as he loses weight and approaches his ideal weight his diabetes improves.

Diabetes which is not controlled by diet alone may be helped by the addition of orally administered hypoglycaemic (blood-sugar lowering) agents such as chlorpropamide and glibenclamide which increase the amount of insulin secreted from the pancreas. The most severe diabetics however need treatment with insulin because their pancreas is incapable of secreting any. Unfortunately if it is given by mouth the hormone is destroyed by acid in the stomach, and hence the only way of administering it is by intramuscular injection once or twice daily. Thus a newly-diagnosed diabetic is admitted to hospital, a suitable diet is worked out for him, and then his insulin requirements are calculated in conjunction with frequent blood and urine tests.

When the patient's blood-sugar level is adequately controlled he is allowed home and subsequently monitors his own progress by testing the amount of sugar in his urine once or twice a day and charting the results.

Diabetes has many complications, for instance, patients with the disorder are prone to arterial disease including ischaemic heart disease, eye disorders causing blindness and disorders of the peripheral nerves causing loss of sensation. There is evidence to suggest that some of these complications may be delayed or avoided by good diabetic control.

The two most important complications of diabetes mellitus from an emergency point of view are both related to the patient's therapy. They are hypoglycaemia (too little sugar in the blood) and hyperglycaemia (too much sugar in the blood). Proper control of diabetes requires the maintenance of a careful balance between three factors, these are:

(1) The amount of food taken in;
(2) The amount of energy expended and
(3) The dose of insulin.

Each diabetic has these values calculated on an individual basis soon after diagnosis, and any variation in one of these three has to be allowed for in the other two. For instance, if a diabetic is off his food for a day or two, as he is taking in less sugar, he will need to reduce his dose of insulin to compensate, otherwise if he sticks to his normal dose, his blood sugar will drop to too low a level (i.e., he will suffer from hypoglycaemia).

However, strict control is very rarely possible and accidents can occur, such as the patient forgetting his insulin altogether one morning or inadvertently giving himself a larger than normal dose.

Hypoglycaemia

This occurs when a patient has either taken too much insulin or too little food and is much more common than hyperglycaemia. The patient's blood-sugar drops and he may feel faint and dizzy, he may start to perspire and if immediate treatment is not given he will become drowsy and finally comatose. Death may follow if proper treatment is not administered. Some patients may become aggressive and appear drunk before losing consciousness and this is one of the many pitfalls which lie open to those who too quickly diagnose drunkeness rather than ascertaining all the facts. The presence of hypoglycaemia can be quickly confirmed by applying a drop of blood, obtained by pricking the ear lobe, to a paper strip which is impregnated with a chemical which changes colour differentially when it is exposed to glucose in blood (Glycemie strips or Dextrostix). The approximate blood-sugar level is obtained and treatment commenced.

Treatment is by the administration of sugar immediately. If the patient is just dizzy and sweaty he can take it in the form of sugar lumps, glucose drinks or very sweet tea/coffee, but if his consciousness is impaired the sugar must be administered i.v. Patients who are drowsy, stuporose or comatose should *never* have drinks forced upon them, as some or all of the fluid may end up in the lungs causing many complications and even death.

Another approach to the reversal of hypoglycaemia is by the

administration of glucagon, this can be given intramuscularly to an unconscious patient and hence may be used by a non-medically trained person (e.g., a member of the patient's family) who can be shown a safe site for intramuscular injection. Its action is nothing like as swift as intravenous glucose but it will help to reverse the fall in blood-sugar.

TABLE 13.1. Contrasting effects of hyperglycaemia and hypoglycaemia

Hypoglycaemia	Hyperglycaemia
Rapid onset	Gradual onset
Conscious level impaired	Conscious level impaired
Moist skin	Dry skin
Normal respiration	Deep rapid breathing with breath smelling of acetone (pear drops)
Tachycardia	Tachycardia

Hyperglycaemia

This occurs when the patient does not take enough insulin or even perhaps forgets to take it at all. Consequently the blood sugar level rises, leading to a more gradual deterioration in the conscious level than in hypoglycaemia. The patient will usually have been unwell for a day or two with nausea, polyuria, polydipsia and he will get gradually drowsier finally becoming comatose.

Diagnosis is established using the impregnated paper sticks (Glycemie strips and Dextrostix) as for hypoglycaemia and treatment consists of an intravenous infusion to correct the patient's dehydration, the correction of any abnormalities in the body chemistry and the initiation of intravenous insulin therapy to reduce the level of blood sugar.

Whilst it is usually a straightforward enough procedure to differentiate between hypo- and hyperglycaemia mistakes can be made unless the level of the sugar in the blood is checked. Insulin should *never* be given to a diabetic who is unwell until his blood-sugar level is known, because if he is already hypoglycaemic you will probably kill him.

Chapter 14

Psychiatric problems

The psychiatrically disturbed can be amongst the most difficult patients to deal with for many reasons, they may vary from the withdrawn and totally inert to, very occasionally, the aggressive and dangerous. Frequently you will see the psychiatric patient when his condition is acute and therefore he is at his most disturbed and agitated. This fact, combined with the apprehension with which 'mad' people are generally viewed means that, in the acute phase, the psychiatric patient is rarely managed correctly outside the environment of a Psychiatric Unit.

When you are called upon to deal with a disturbed patient try and remember the following points:

(1) A relaxed, quiet, objective approach is vital.
(2) Anxiety and aggression in a patient tends to produce the same reactions in you. If you do not completely control these feelings the situation rapidly deteriorates.
(3) When you are apprehensive and annoyed, remember that in a difficult and unfamiliar situation, your judgment may be clouded. When you can, do not make snap decisions, count to twenty and think again.
(4) Always talk to the patient. Even if you are inexperienced in handling such events, discussing his situation with him helps. Silence only serves to increase tension, so use your common sense and indulge in supportive discussion.

Specific psychiatric disorders

Schizophrenia

This is a condition in which the patient tends to withdraw into himself and his thinking becomes confused and disordered. He may be deluded and feel he is being persecuted, (this is known as paranoia) or hallucinated. The hallucination may take the form of the patient hearing voices (auditory hallucinations) or having visions (visual hallucinations).

It is understandable that these disturbances can result in very bizarre behaviour particularly when the patient is in the acute phase of the disease. Under these circumstances the patient is usually admitted to a Psychiatric Unit, where he is treated with one of the Phenothiazine group of drugs, e.g., chlorpromazine (Largactil).

The acute attack is unfortunately frequently followed by a chronic phase with the patient continuing on treatment, now in the form of depot injections (injections which are given once a month and which slowly release the active drug into the blood stream over this period). In this phase he is often quiet and withdrawn sometimes exhibiting mildly 'eccentric' behaviour. Further acute exacerbations may however occur, and the condition is only rarely 'cured' completely.

Depression and mania

These are disorders of mood with depression being far more common than mania. A patient who is depressed appears permanently sad, complains of a lack of interest in everything and of having no energy. There is an inability to sleep, and a loss of appetite amongst other things. This depression may occur in response to a personal tragedy for the patient, (e.g., the death of a close relative), and this type of depression is known as reactive depression in that the patient's depressed mood is a reaction to the sad event.

On the other hand depression may arise for no known reason and under these circumstances it is known as endogenous depression.

The treatment of depression is via the use of certain drugs known as antidepressants, e.g., mianserin (Bolvidon) and also via electroconvulsive therapy (ECT). ECT consists of giving the anaesthetized patient a small electric shock to the brain which can, in certain patients, improve the condition.

Mania occurs only very occasionally, and manic patients tend to be inordinately cheerful, a permanent 'life and soul of the party'. The patient maintains this mood even when it is totally inappropriate, he will chatter on interminably and is hyperactive moving from one activity to another but rarely completing any task. Treatment is via mild tranquillizers and sedatives.

Anxiety

A patient with this disorder is permanently anxious or apprehensive, sometimes having acute attacks on top of a chronic basic condition. It is found most commonly in the adolescent and the aged who worry about such things as their health or what their future holds. Treatment is by the use of such tranquillizers as lorazepam (Ativan).

Dementia

In this condition a person experiences a slow but persistent deterioration in his intellectual capacity, gradually becoming mentally incompetent and almost child-like again. The whole process is irreversible and commonly occurs due to narrowing of the arteries supplying blood and hence oxygen to the brain.

Chapter 15

Poisoning

Poisoning may be accidental or deliberate, the latter being the more common. The poison itself may be taken in by any one of four different routes, these are:

(1) Ingestion
(2) Inhalation
(3) Injection
(4) Absorption

Ingestion

Food poisoning

Under these circumstances the patient or patients have all eaten the same meal, which has turned out to be contaminated by bacteria, usually one of the Salmonella species. This commonly results in the sudden onset of acute colicky abdominal pain associated with diarrhoea and vomiting.

The majority of cases improve quite quickly as they are fairly mild, some need no drug treatment at all whilst others settle after just a few days symptomatic therapy with or without antibiotics.

Unfortunately, however, the very young, the very old and the debilitated are more at risk, and acute collapse and death can and do occur amongst these categories of patients.

Paediatric

Young children will put almost anything in their mouths and often subsequently swallow it. Sometimes they are lucky and the substances are innocuous, on other occasions this is not the case. The possible list of poisons is endless and includes drugs prescribed for relatives, household and cosmetic items, seeds and berries, etc.

Deliberate self-poisoning

Unfortunately, this is very common. The usual patient is a female in the 15–30 age group who is making a not very serious attempt on her life. Whilst in many of these patients the attempt may be felt to be frivolous, in others it must be regarded as a warning of a significant underlying psychiatric or personal problem. These latter patients need help, as if their cry is ignored it may lead to a second, more serious and possibly successful attempt at self-destruction.

Inhalation

Injury and death can result from the inhalation of toxic fumes or gases. This may be accidental, for instance where a person is asleep in a poorly ventilated room in which there is a badly installed gas heater, or a deliberate attempt at suicide.

The commonest way of attempting suicide by inhalation is to sit in a car in a locked garage with the engine running, the resultant inhalation of the carbon monoxide rendering the patient unconscious and finally asphyxiating him.

Injection

Poisoning by injection can occur by accident, when a person is bitten by a poisonous animal, e.g., an adder or viper. This is very rare in the United Kingdom but occurs more frequently in countries where poisonous snakes are common, e.g., India and Burma.

Drug addicts who 'main line', i.e., administer the drugs on which they are dependent directly into the vein, are very prone to accidental over-dosage as they are often unaware exactly what dose they are receiving.

Absorption

A very few substances, e.g., some very toxic herbicides and insecticides can be absorbed through unbroken skin and will cause serious illness and even death when taken in quite small amounts. This type of problem is seen in people who are inadvertently exposed to the chemical, when for instance, crops are being sprayed or dusted from a light aeroplane.

Management of the poisoned patient

The management of the poisoned patient may be divided into three phases:

(1) Initial resuscitative measures.
(2) An attempt to limit the amount of poison entering the blood stream.
(3) Specific treatment to counteract the effect of the drug and measures to treat any complications that may occur.

Initial resuscitation

As many poisoned patients have an impairment of consciousness the maintenance of an open airway has a high priority.

If the patient is shocked an attempt must be made to maintain the blood supply to the brain and other essential organs by lying the patient flat or even tipping him head down and elevating his legs.

Always be alert for a respiratory arrest as certain drugs, e.g., opiates and barbiturates, depress respiration grossly.

Observe and note the patient's vital signs (pulse, respiration level of consciousness, pupil responses).

Having stabilized the patient's condition now attempt to find out:

(1) What poison has been administered?
(2) By what route?
(3) How much?
(4) When?
(5) Whether taken with alcohol?

Any information you gain must accompany the patient to the hospital together with other facts which may be of use.

Minimization of blood levels

Ingestion

Ingested poisons rest for a short while in the stomach where some absorption takes place. They then pass into the small intestine where the rest of the drug is absorbed. There are four ways in which the blood levels may be kept low, these are:

(1) By emptying the stomach as quickly as possible after the drug has been ingested. This is carried out in one of two ways, either by gastric lavage or by the induction of an emesis (vomiting).

Gastric lavage (stomach washout) consists of the flushing out of that structure's contents by the passage of a wide bore plastic tube through the mouth, down the oesophagus and into the stomach.

Several litres of water are then poured down the tube following which the fluid is drained out again hopefully together with any of the poison which remained in the stomach.

An emesis is produced by giving the patient an emetic (i.e. a drug which induces vomiting) e.g., syrup of ipecacuanha. This makes the patient vomit up the poison which remains in his stomach.

Both of these manoeuvres should only be carried out *in hospital*. *Do not* dose a patient with some supposed emetic, e.g., strongly salted water, as you will only make his condition worse.

Never attempt to make a patient with an impairment of consciousness drink anything, as it will usually run into his lungs rather than his stomach and you will drown him.

(2) By adsorbing the drug in the small intestine and thus preventing its absorption into the blood stream. This is done by administering orally substances, such as activated charcoal, which attach themselves to the poison when they get into the gut, and thus prevent its absorption into the blood stream. Unfortunately, this does not work for all poisons but can be usefully employed in, for instance, poisoning by certain of the antidepressants.

(3) By 'hurrying' the poison through the gut. This may be achieved by administering a purgative to the patient, and as the poison is 'hurried' through the intestine there is less time for it to be absorbed.

(4) By increasing the rate at which the drug, if it has already been absorbed into the blood stream, is excreted. Certain drugs, e.g., aspirin are excreted in the urine and if the production of urine is increased by the use of diuretics and intravenous infusions the level of drug in the blood can be made to drop more rapidly.

Sometimes renal dialysis may be used for exactly the same reason.

Inhalation

The amount of gas breathed in may be minimized by removing the patient from the gas-filled room as rapidly as possible *given that it is safe to do so*.

Nothing is to be gained by you rushing straight into the danger area and being overcome by fumes whilst struggling to remove an unconscious patient.

Remember *safety first*. Try and cut off the flow of gas, then get fresh air into the room by opening the windows or doors or if absolutely necessary smashing the windows.

Where available use breathing apparatus and make sure you have at least one companion outside the danger area who has you on a safety line. Immediately the patient is out administer oxygen having ensured an open airway.

Injection

When a snake bites, venom is injected beneath the skin, it causes local damage in the bitten area and also is slowly absorbed into the blood stream directly, and indirectly via the lymphatic channels. It is not the local effects which kill the patient but the systemic effects when the poison attacks organs such as the heart and central nervous system.

The immediate treatment of a snake bite is to calm the patient, lie him down and put a dry dressing over the bite. Where a limb is involved, a crepe bandage should be applied firmly (*not* as a tourniquet) and the limb kept elevated above the level of the heart. These measures will all help to minimize the absorption of venom into the blood stream.

Absorption

Where a patient has been contaminated by a substance which is absorbed directly through the skin it is essential to remove the contaminated clothing and wash the patient down thoroughly.

Do remember when you are considering this course of action that you must not get yourself contaminated.

Specific treatment

Certain drugs have specific antagonists which reverse their most dangerous effects. For instance the opiate group which include heroin and morphine can cause severe respiratory depression which is reversed by the substances known as nalorphine (Narcan). This is given intravenously and can very quickly revive a moribund patient.

Unfortunately however, such specific and effective remedies are rarely available and most drugs do not have good antidotes.

The complications which occur secondary to poisoning are many and varied and include such things as respiratory depression, shock, liver failure, convulsions, cardiac arrhythmias, etc. These are all treated appropriately as they arise.

Drugs commonly used in self-poisoning

Benzodiazepines   The many members of this large group of drugs are used mainly as hypnotics and tranquillizers, e.g. fluorazepam (Dalmane), nitrazepam (Mogadon), diazepam (Valium), lorazepam (Ativan). Generally speaking these drugs are very safe and do not kill even when taken in large doses.

Paracetamol   This is a dangerous drug to take in large doses as it can cause, amongst other things, fatal liver damage. It may be found not only as straightforward paracetamol tablets but also in combination with other drugs, e.g. with dextropropoxyphene in Distalgesic. Several proprietary analgesics which are available without prescription also contain the drug.

Aspirin   Overdoses of aspirin can be fatal due to the acute upset they cause in the body chemistry. As with paracetamol the drug may be found alone or as a combination tablet, many of the latter being available without prescription.

Antidepressants   There are several different groups of drugs which have an anti-depressant action. These include lithium, the mono amine oxidase inhibitors, tricyclics and tetracyclics. In overdose they can have serious effects on the heart and blood pressure.

Opiates   Drugs of the opiate group, e.g., heroin, morphine, pethidine, cause respiratory depression and arrest, and overdoses are nearly always associated with narcotic abuse.

A complication of many overdoses is that the tablets are often washed down with alcohol which potentiates the drug taken thus making the overdose much more serious.

Chapter 16

Fractures

A fracture is an interruption in the continuity of a bone which can either be cracked, broken, splintered, chipped or buckled.

Causes of fractures

Fractures can occur secondary to direct force or indirect force.

Direct force

Here damage to the bone occurs at the point at which the force is applied, e.g., a kick on the shin resulting in a fractured tibia.

Indirect force

In this instance damage to the bone occurs at a point some distance away from the area of the blow, for example a fractured clavicle can sometimes be caused where a patient tries to save himself from falling by taking the impact on the outstretched hand. The force of the blow on the hand is transmitted up the stiff arm and fractures the clavicle.

There are two other types of fractures which occur occasionally, first, the pathological fracture where the bone breaks as a result of having been weakened by a disease process, e.g., osteoporosis (page 116). Under these conditions fractures can occur with minimal force, for instance a patient who slips off a low chair onto a thickly carpeted floor can fracture the neck of her femur. The second type is due to muscular action, when damage to the bone occurs secondary to a sudden, unexpected and violent contraction of the attached muscles, for example if a patient receives an electric shock, sudden spasm of the arm muscles can result in a fracture of one of the bones in the limb.

Types of fracture

(1) Closed fracture – where there is no break in the skin surrounding the site of the fracture. (*See Figure 16.1 (a) and (b)*).

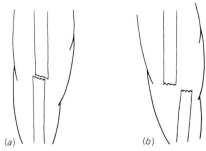

(a)   (b)

Figure 16.1a Slightly displaced closed fracture
Figure 16.1b Grossly displaced closed fracture

(2) Open fracture – where there is a break in the continuity of the skin surrounding the site of the fracture allowing air and bacteria to enter. The jagged ends of the bone may appear through the skin and this type of injury is also known as a compound fracture (*see Figure 16.2*).

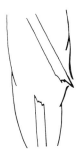

Figure 16.2 Open (Compound) fracture

Either type of fracture may be *complicated* by injury to structures other than bones, e.g., spleen, lungs, blood vessels or nerves, which lie near the fracture.

When the bone is shattered into several pieces the fracture is known as a comminuted one (*see Figure 16.3*).

Where the broken ends of the bone are jammed back firmly together by the force of the fall, the fracture is said to be impacted (*see Figure 16.4*).

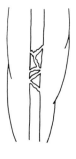

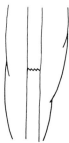

Figure 16.3 Comminuted fracture

Figure 16.4 Impacted fracture

In children, whose bones are less brittle than those of adults, a special type of fracture occurs which is known as a greenstick fracture. Under these circumstances the bone tends to buckle rather than break completely (*see Figure 16.5*).

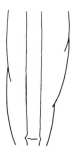

Figure 16.5 Greenstick fracture

Assessment of a fracture

The history of the accident will give you some idea as to how likely it is that the patient has fractured a bone.

Clinical features indicating a fracture

Loss of power and control

The casualty is unable to move and control the affected part normally and cannot prevent any unnatural movement.

Swelling and bruising

This is due to blood loss into the surrounding tissues, the amount of swelling being an indication of the amount of blood loss.

Deformity

The affected part often appears to be mis-shapen, perhaps rotated, angulated or shortened.

Irregularity

The surface of the bone as it is felt beneath the skin may have a bump or a sharp edge, though sometimes the amount of swelling present may disguise this.

Unnatural movement

At the site of the fracture a 'false joint' has been created and movement may occur at this site.

Crepitus

This refers to the grating which may be heard and felt as the broken ends of the bone rub against each other on movement of the injured limb. This is a sign which should never be deliberately sought but may be noted accidentally whilst you are supporting or immobilizing the injured limb.

Always compare the injured and uninjured sides.

The patient will complain of pain around the fracture site which is increased by movement of the injured limb and gentle pressure to the affected area causes pain.

Treatment

General treatment

If possible treat the fracture where the injury occurred before moving the casualty, unless it is obviously dangerous to do so.

Support the affected part of the body to prevent further movement until it is satisfactorily immobilized.

Immobilize the fracture as appropriate with splints remembering that this must include the joint above and below the fracture whilst you try to avoid any direct pressure on the fracture site. Check at 10 minute intervals to ensure that the splinting is not becoming too tight on the limb as it swells following the injury. The constriction that can result will impede the circulation of blood down the limb and may permanently damage it.

Check the integrity of the circulation in the affected limb by examining the colour and temperature of the skin distal to the fracture. Also check for the presence of a pulse in this area before and after treatment.

Check the skin sensation in the area distal to the fracture before and after treatment. Also ask the patient about the presence of any tingling or numbness in the injured limb.

A deformity in a fractured limb may occasionally need to be corrected urgently, if for instance the circulation down the limb is impaired. Where possible the correction should be undertaken in hospital under general anaesthetic.

Entonox should be offered to the patient to relieve pain if this is significant.

The injured limb where possible should be elevated in order to reduce the swelling.

Where you are dealing with an open fracture, expose the injury in a good light, but of course keep movement of the limb to a minimum. If necessary cut away clothing and then place sterile dressings on each side of the wound, building them up around the fracture to form a bridge. Keep the wound as clean as possible whilst avoiding direct pressure onto it. Check your dressing and the limb at regular intervals (10 minutes). It is important that open fractures are kept as uncontaminated as possible, as if the bone becomes infected (osteomyelitis) the patient's recovery will be seriously delayed.

Splints

Splints should be long enough and firm enough to immobilize the joint above and below the fracture and should be wide enough to provide full support for the limb. They should be well padded so that they are comfortable and should be placed on the limb outside the patient's clothing.

Splinting a fracture immobilizes it and thus prevents movement of the broken ends of the bone, reducing pain and preventing further damage to the surrounding tissues.

Treatment of specific fractures

As a general rule most fractures of the upper limb can be supported and immobilized by the use of a sling and/or using body bandages to secure the limb to the trunk. Fractures of the lower limb may be supported and immobilized by splinting the injured and uninjured limbs together.

Clavicle

Place a soft pad in the axilla and support the arm of the injured side in a triangular sling, then secure the limb to the chest with a broad triangular body bandage or frac-strap over the sling.

Scapula

Place the patient in a sitting position and support the arm of the injured side in a broad arm sling.

Humerus

Place a soft pad in the axilla and support the arm in a broad arm sling. A body bandage may be needed to secure the limb to the chest.

Forearm

A pneumatic splint is useful for immobilizing such an injury together with a broad arm sling.

Hand

The hand should be supported in a high sling to reduce swelling.

Elbow

This may be supported in a broad arm sling or a collar and cuff and may be secured to the chest with bandages or frac-straps. Do not attempt to force the elbow to bend or straighten. Allow it to rest in the most comfortable position.

Spine

Movement of a patient with a spinal injury should be minimal so when you arrive on site instruct the patient to lie quite still.

Do not turn the casualty. Assess, treat and subsequently load the patient in the position in which he was found.

Steady and support the head, (*see Figure 16.6*) shoulders and pelvis and pad between the legs. Secure the ankles and feet using a figure-of-eight, and secure the knees and thighs with broad triangular bandages or wide frac-straps.

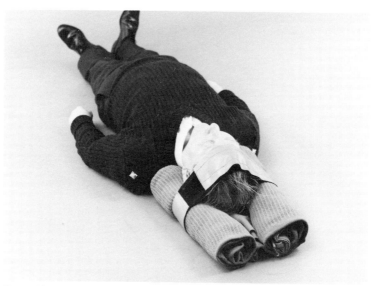

Figure 16.6 Head and neck supported using a blanket and frac-strap.

A cervical collar must always be used when an injury to the cervical region is suspected. This will also aid in the maintenance of an open airway.

Transfer the patient to a cot with the minimum of movement, preferably using a scoop stretcher, (*see* p. 206). If you are placing the casualty on a cot in the supine position, spinal support pads should be placed under the neck and the small of the back.

Ribs

Rib fractures are dealt with in the chapter on Chest Injuries.

Pelvis

Pad well between the legs and secure the ankles and feet with a figure-of-eight using either a triangular bandage or a long frac-strap. The knee joints should be secured with the use of a broad triangular bandage or a frac-strap. The pelvis may be supported using three folded triangular bandages, broad frac-straps or a roll of towel or a folded blanket.

Femur

A fractured femur must be immobilized above the pelvis and below the knee, (*see Figure 16.7*) therefore a well padded long splint is placed on the outer side of the leg, extending from the axilla to beyond the foot of the injured limb with a short well padded splint between the legs. These splints should be secured by triangular bandages or frac-straps.

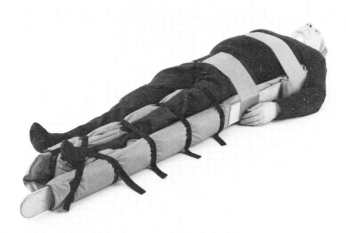

Figure 16.7 Completed splint for a fractured femur.

Tibia and fibula

Fractures in this region may be immobilized well using pneumatic splints (*see Figure 16.8*) or perhaps two well padded splints, one each side of the injured limb, secured by bandages or frac-straps (*see Figure 16.9*).

Ankle and foot

Do not remove the shoe unless bleeding is suspected. Fractures in the

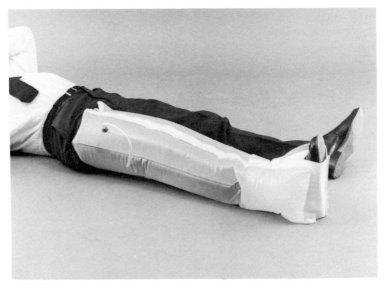

Figure 16.8 Pneumatic splint supporting a fracture of the tibia and fibula.

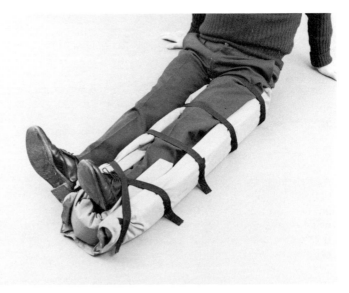

Figure 16.9 Splinting of fractured tibia and fibula. Note the well padded splints applied over clothing.

region may be treated by short pneumatic splints or a rolled blanket made up in the shape of a stirrup secured by triangular bandages or frac-straps.

Dislocations

A dislocation is the displacement from their normal position of one or more of the bones of a joint (*see Figure 16.10*). This alone results in the joint becoming useless though dislocations may also be accompanied by a fracture, the so-called fracture-dislocation.

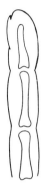 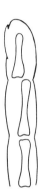

Figure 16.10 A dislocation. The finger on the left is normal, the one on the right shows a dislocation at the inter-phalangeal joint.

The clinical features of a dislocation resemble those of a fracture, with pain at the site of the injury, deformity, and immobility.

Commonly dislocated joints are those of the fingers and also the shoulder joint.

The treatment for dislocation is to immobilize the joint in the position in which it is found and not to attempt to correct the deformity, (i.e. not to *reduce* the dislocation).

Sprains

A sprain is the over-stretching and tearing of the ligaments and tissues around a joint. The joint most commonly affected is the ankle which swells up, becomes bruised and is painful to move or to walk on. A severe sprain can be difficult to distinguish from a fracture and if in doubt regard it as a fracture until proven otherwise.

Treatment for a sprain consists of rest and support of the injured joint with ample soft padding held in place by a crepe bandage. A cold compress is sometimes useful in the acute stage to ease pain and to reduce the swelling.

Hospital treatment of fractures

Most fractures mend satisfactorily, if treated properly, though they do take months to heal rather than the week or so that a straightforward skin laceration would need. The treatment of most limb fractures consists of the immobilization of the correctly aligned bony fragments in the normal anatomical position. The immobilization is achieved and maintained by the use of a plaster of Paris splint which is kept in place for some weeks/months. For instance in the case of an uncomplicated fracture of the radius the cast would remain on for about five weeks, where with a straightforward fracture of the tibia it would need to remain in place for up to 8 weeks.

Sometimes, where a fracture is badly comminuted, the patient may need to be operated upon and the bones fixed together by means of screws and plates. These fastenings are allowed to remain in place until the fracture is securely united, and then may be removed.

Chapter 17

Injuries to head and face

Head injuries

Head injuries are common and vary in severity from a blow which leaves one transiently dazed to one which kills instantly. Damage can occur to the scalp (bruising or a laceration), to the skull (a fracture), to the blood vessels inside the skull (these can be ruptured and thus bleed compressing the brain), or to the brain itself (which can be bruised or lacerated).

Specific injuries

Scalp wounds

Bleeding from scalp wounds is often profuse and as the wound cannot be seen, the patient, especially if a child, may become very distressed by the sight of blood on his hands and running down his face. It can be very difficult to locate the exact site and the extent of the wound, due to matting of the hair around the area by blood, and for a proper assessment of the wound and its subsequent suturing it is often necessary to shave the hair on that part of the head. The majority of scalp wounds just need cleaning and suturing though of course occasionally they may cover an underlying skull fracture.

Skull fractures

Fractures of the skull may be open or closed and are associated with injuries to the brain and sometimes with damage to the cervical spine. The fracture may be to the vault or to the base of the skull, and occasionally vault fractures are depressed. A depressed fracture is one in which the blow has been sufficient to push the broken fragments of skull inwards, thus leaving a dent on the surface of the head where the bones are *depressed* and press on the surface of the brain.

Fractures of the base of the skull may be suspected when any or all of the following physical signs are noted:

(1) The patient has a 'black eye' with no evidence of external injury to the orbit, cheek bones or nose.
(2) When CSF or a mixture of blood and CSF is seen to be leaking down the nostril.
(3) When CSF or a mixture of blood and CSF is leaking out of the ear.

Whilst the majority of skull fractures are closed, open fractures do occur and are dangerous in that they allow micro-organisms such as bacteria, direct access to the intracranial cavity.

Bleeding inside the skull

Underlying the skull and surrounding the brain are numerous blood vessels. Should the head injury be sufficiently severe to cause one or more of these to rupture bleeding occurs into the closed box of the skull. As this bleeding continues, the brain becomes subject to more and more *compression*, by this slowly enlarging haematoma (*see Figure 17.1*). Furthermore the damage that the brain itself has suffered secondary to the blow, causes it to swell (cerebral oedema) a factor which merely worsens the situation.

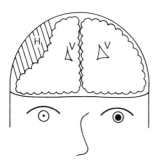

Figure 17.1 Diagrammatic illustration of compression of brain produced by bleeding into skull following a head injury. Note the unequal pupils, which may be dilated on the injured side or constricted as illustrated here, the pattern being variable: H = Haematoma; V = Cerebral Ventricles.

Patients who have sustained an injury of sufficient severity to produce such a haematoma will probably have suffered an episode of unconsciousness. They may subsequently recover consciousness but often go on to become drowsy, then stuporose and finally comatose again, as the pressure inside the skull builds up with continued bleeding.

Other signs of an intracranial haematoma are abnormalities in the pupils, for instance instead of being equal in size, one may be larger than the other (dilated) and poorly responsive to light, and weakness of the limbs on one side of the body together perhaps with abnormalities of speech and the occurrence of convulsions. There may be a bradycardia and the patient's respiration may be stertorous (noisy/snoring).

As the intracranial pressure increases so the patient's condition deteriorates until eventually death supervenes. Investigation is urgently required to locate the site of the haematoma and this is normally done using a CAT scanner. Following this, drill holes (burr holes) are made over the area and the haematoma drained with, if possible, the bleeding vessel being tied off.

Brain damage

Brain damage occurs due to three factors:

(1) The blow itself can cause bruising and laceration to the brain.
(2) As the brain is shaken about inside the skull, it is bruised by coming into violent contact with the hard inner surface of that bony box.
(3) If as was described in the previous paragraph, blood vessels inside the skull rupture and bleed, the resultant compression produces further brain damage.

The severity of the injury will vary widely, but any significant head injury will inevitably result in some degree of brain damage even though this may be minor. The damage is cumulative and repeated head injuries can result in the patient becoming totally incapacitated. For instance, in boxers who receive frequent blows to the head, should they have a long boxing career in which they are often knocked out they will end up 'punch drunk' as their brains are irreversibly damaged.

The cardinal syndrome seen in a person who has suffered a head injury is *concussion*. The features of concussion are:

(1) A head injury which has jarred the brain and produced
(2) Some impairment of consciousness however transient. The patient will often
(3) Feel nauseated and indeed may vomit. Particularly where children are involved they may subsequently
(4) Become drowsy and want to be left alone to sleep. Not infrequently the concussed patient also exhibits some degree of
(5) Amnesia for the events surrounding the incident. This may be pre-traumatic, (i.e., he may have forgotten some of the events leading up to the accident), post-traumatic, (i.e., although he was unconscious for only a matter of 4–5 minutes he will not

remember anything that happened for 4–5 hours after his accident), or both. Finally and most commonly, he will complain of
(6) Headache, which is usually generalized rather than being related to the area of the head on which he was struck.

Not all of these features are necessarily present in all patients with head injuries, and whilst the amnesia tends to be permanent, the other features disappear fairly quickly, though the headaches can recur intermittently for some months.

Treatment of head injuries

(1) Be alert for possible injuries to the cervical spine.
(2) Where there is an impairment of consciousness, safe-guard the airway.
(3) Treat any significant bleeding from the head or elsewhere.
(4) Thoroughly examine the patient and then if appropriate put into the three-quarter prone position with the injured side of the head downwards.
(5) Oxygen should be administered and the patient's vital signs monitored and recorded.
(6) On arrival at hospital, X-rays of the skull and cervical spine will be necessary and if there is any suspicion of an intracranial haematoma, CAT scanning.

Facial injuries

Facial injuries can appear very alarming to the person who is aiding the casualty, and be extremely distressing to the patient himself. Bleeding is usually profuse and swelling of tissues around the eyes often causes visual problems, whilst damage to the nose and mouth can produce some airway obstruction and difficulty in communication.

Specific injuries

Nose

The nose when damaged bleeds briskly and swells making breathing difficult. Sometimes a fracture is obvious due to the extent of the displacement, however, often the amount of swelling present can mask this. If badly displaced the nasal bones will need to be manipulated under anaesthetic in order to regain an acceptable appearance. Leakage of CSF down the nose indicates a fracture of the base of the skull.

Eyes

The eyes themselves may be damaged, e.g., puncture wounds, etc. or may be affected by damage to the bony walls of the orbit.

Cheek bones

The bones of the cheek are hollow and fracture quite easily, with fragments of bone being pushed inwards (depressed). This depression may be obvious visually or easily detected when the cheeks are gently touched. The pieces of bone will need to be elevated at operation.

Mandible

This is commonly injured in assaults and the victim complains of pain in the jaw particularly on movement, so that speaking, chewing and swallowing are difficult. He will also feel that his teeth do not meet properly when he closes his jaw, this being due to the displacement which inevitably takes place.

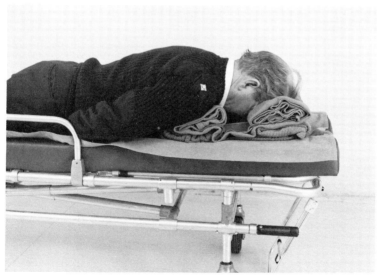

Figure 17.2 Positioning for a patient who is unconscious, with severe facial injuries.

Treatment of facial injuries

(1) Safe-guard the airway as bleeding takes place inside the nose and mouth and blood clots can cause blockages. This is particularly important when there is an associated impairment of consciousness.
(2) Remove false or detached teeth.
(3) Where the patient is conscious sit him forward so that blood drips outwards into a receiver rather than inwards into the airway.
(4) If the lower jaw is damaged this should be supported.
(5) Where there is severe damage or unconsciousness and bleeding, the patient may need to be lain prone, supported by blankets at the head and chest leaving a well in between these into which blood or vomit may drain (*see Figure 17.2*).
(6) It is important to remember that injuries to the face may be accompanied by damage to the brain, skull and cervical spine.

Chapter 18

Injuries to the abdomen

Injuries to the abdomen may be divided into two categories. Firstly, closed (non-penetrating) and secondly open (penetrating). The major problem connected with either type of injury is the possibility that one of the intra-abdominal organs, e.g. liver/kidney/spleen may have been damaged with consequent bleeding which can be severe.

Closed (non-penetrating) injuries

These are the more common in the United Kingdom and need careful assessment, as damage can be caused to any or all of the intra-abdominal viscera.

The solid organs

A blow to the abdomen landing either in the region of the liver or the spleen can lacerate the underlying organ, whilst the kidneys tend to be damaged more frequently by blows which land in the loin rather than the anterior part of the abdominal wall. Bleeding from a damaged kidney can result in haematuria, whilst bleeding into the peritoneal cavity from lacerations to the liver or spleen causes abdominal pain as blood is extremely irritant to the peritoneum. The patient's abdomen may be rigid to the touch as he is 'guarding' the damaged intra-abdominal structures by keeping his abdominal musculature tensed. If the bleeding continues at significant levels the patient's blood pressure will fall and his pulse rate rise until he eventually becomes shocked, and unless surgery is undertaken to arrest the blood-loss death will inevitably result.

The injuries to the solid organs may be minor ones which bleed slightly and then quickly stop, under which circumstances they are usually never definitely diagnosed as no treatment is needed. However, if they are more severe and bleeding is significant, operative intervention is needed and the lacerations have to be repaired surgically. Sometimes repair is not possible and the whole of a ruptured spleen may need to be removed (splenectomy) or perhaps part of a lacerated liver (partial hepatectomy). The spleen may be removed completely as survival is possible without it, however life is not sustainable without a liver and hence as much as possible of that structure must be preserved.

The hollow structures

A severe blow to the abdomen may cause any of the following hollow structures to rupture:

The major blood vessels

For example, the aorta or inferior vena cava. If one of these vessels is torn, bleeding is usually catastrophic, the patient quickly becoming shocked and dying.

The gut

Rupture of the gut causes leakage of the contents which will soil the peritoneum and produce peritonitis. Such damage requires surgical intervention to close the laceration and clean the peritoneal cavity.

The bladder

Urine will leak from a ruptured bladder and again immediate closure of the defect is necessary.

The diaphragm

This thin sheet of muscle which separates the abdominal cavity from the thoracic cavity can be ruptured secondary to abdominal trauma. This may result in herniation of abdominal contents, e.g., stomach, through the hole in the diaphragm into the chest. Again this is a condition which needs rapid repair.

Open (penetrating) injuries

Open injuries may be caused by knives, shards of broken glass, gunshot wounds, etc. They are, in the United Kingdom, at least, much less common than the non-penetrating type. For the correct management of a case it is always important to know what type of instrument has caused the injury so that some kind of assessment may be made as to what depth of penetration has occurred. For preference the instrument should accompany the patient to hospital.

All entry and exit wounds should be noted, do not forget that the patient may have been stabbed more than once and the sites of the wounds will give you some idea as to what structures may be involved, e.g., an entry wound in the right hypochondrium can result in a laceration of the liver.

The majority of patients with penetrating wounds will need surgery in order to inspect the contents of the abdominal cavity, repair any damage, and clean the soiled peritoneum.

In a few cases not only will there be an incised wound in the abdominal wall but also some of the contents of the abdomen will have spilled out through the wound, this usually being the small intestine. Under these circumstances surgical repair is of course mandatory, however no attempt should be made to replace the intestines prior to surgery as unnecessary handling of the gut always damages it. Further, replacing it prematurely will inevitably soil the peritoneum to a greater extent than has occurred already. Both of these factors will lead to an increased incidence of complications such as peritonitis and thus endanger the life of the patient. Until the patient is in the operating theatre, the spilled gut should be kept covered with a clean (sterile if possible) sheet and receive the minimum of handling.

Investigation of abdominal injuries

X-ray of chest, abdomen and pelvis are necessary together with an estimation of the patient's haemoglobin level in an attempt to get a rough idea of blood loss, if any. A urine sample must be obtained to check for haematuria and sometimes it is necessary to insert a needle into the abdominal cavity in order to ascertain if bleeding has taken place into that space. Where renal damage is suspected the patient should have an IVP.

Chapter 19

Injuries to the chest

The immediately critical problem with an injury to the chest is that the patient's respiration may be jeopardized consequent upon the damage sustained. The second urgent problem is that with the heart and major blood vessels situated within the thorax there may be a laceration of one of these resulting in a major loss of blood.

As with injuries to the abdomen we may divide chest injuries into penetrating and non-penetrating types. The latter are by far the more common in the United Kingdom.

Closed (non-penetrating) injuries

The majority of such injuries are inconsequential with the damage usually being confined to bruising to the musculature of the chest wall, sometimes accompanied by a fracture to one or perhaps two ribs and with no significant damage to the underlying heart/lungs. This type of injury is common secondary to such things as sporting activities (blow/kick to the chest), perhaps an accident at work or in the home, where the patient strikes his chest against a table or work-bench, having slipped.

However, more significant injuries can occur, particularly secondary to road traffic accidents, where the patients suffer multiple rib fractures which may be complicated by associated damage to the heart/great vessels or lungs.

Superficial bruising

This is inconsequential and the patient will only need treatment with analgesics.

Fractured rib

The patient's chest is tender on palpation over the site of the fracture and he is in continuous pain in the acute stages, the pain being made worse by deep breathing or coughing (ie pleuritic chest pain). An X-ray will reveal the fracture and treatment is simple consisting of support for the arm on the injured side in a broad arm sling and administration of analgesics.

The jagged end of a fractured rib may occasionally pierce the underlying lung and cause it to deflate producing a pneumothorax, this will need treatment as discussed on page 34. Occasionally also a significant amount of bleeding may occur into the pleural space around the lung (C.F. pleural effusion, page 32). As the 'effusion' is made up of blood it is known as a *haemothorax* and as with a pleural effusion it may need drainage. Where bleeding occurs into the lung as the result of an injury the patient may cough up blood (haemoptysis) which always alarms him, but if secondary to a minor injury is not usually anything to worry about.

Multiple rib fractures

Whilst fracture of a single rib or even of two or three is painful and distressing to the patient it is not, in the vast majority of cases, a major medical problem. However, where there are multiple rib fractures the patient's life may well be in jeopardy, as the bellows mechanism of the chest is disrupted and the patient is unable to properly inhale or exhale.

Where a patient has been, for instance, involved in a serious road traffic accident (RTA), and struck in the chest by the steering wheel, three or four ribs may have been broken in more than one place (*see Figure 19.1*) the result being that one segment of the

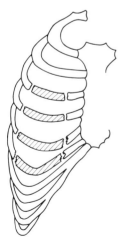

Figure 19.1 Diagrammatic representation of a hemi-thorax with a flail segment (cross hatched) involving four ribs.

ribcage, (i.e., the bellows) is detached from the main part. This is known as a 'flail segment' and the condition is sometimes called a stove-in-chest.

Normally as the patient is respiring the whole chest expands during inspiration and contracts on expiration, however, where there is a flail segment, this portion of the chest wall does exactly the opposite, i.e. when the patient inspires, the flail-segment falls inwards and when he expires it moves outwards. This total disruption of the normal mechanism means that the patient is gasping for breath, probably cyanosed and certainly very agitated. 'Paradoxical' movement of the flail segment and the bruising which is often present in the underlying lung result in a degree of oxygen lack, and treatment is aimed towards temporarily stabilizing the segment as soundly as possible to ensure that the patient reaches hospital alive where definitive treatment may be carried out. Movement of the flail segment is minimized by padding the area and lying the patient on the injured side perhaps with the arm strapped across the chest. Pressure is thus applied and stabilizes the flail segment. Where the injury is central and anterior involving the sternum, something bulky such as a pillow may be strapped across the front of the chest aiding the stability of the detached area.

When the patient is admitted to hospital, if the segment is a significant one and is seriously affecting his respiration, his breathing will be taken over by a machine (a ventilator). Operation may later be necessary to wire together the broken ends of the ribs.

Injuries to the heart and great vessels

Occasionally severe blunt trauma to the chest (e.g., RTAs) can result in damage to the heart and great vessels. If the aorta or left ventricle are torn open death is inevitable and usually rapid. If however the tear in the aorta is only through part of the wall and not the whole thickness, the structure dilates and forms an aneurysm. This will be seen on X-ray and will need to be repaired urgently as the tear may subsequently extend and the aorta rupture completely.

Rupture of the diaphragm

This topic is discussed in the Chapter on Injuries to the Abdomen.

Open (penetrating) injuries

These are commonly secondary to stab wounds and can result in a pneumothorax or a haemothorax. Very rarely air may be heard being sucked into the chest through a wound as a patient inspires and if you examine the area some of the air will be noted bubbling out again when he breathes out. This is called a 'sucking' chest wound and the immediate treatment is to place a firm dressing over the wound to prevent air being drawn in. The wound can then be explored and later properly closed when the patient arrives at the hospital.

Obviously stab wounds to the thorax can sever blood vessels and if the patient is unfortunate enough to have a major artery cut, death can ensue rapidly. The definitive treatment for such an injury is urgent surgery in order to ligate the severed vessel.

Wherever possible, when a patient with a penetrating chest wound is admitted the implement which has caused the wound should accompany him together with as detailed a history of the injury as is available.

Investigation of chest injuries

The most important investigation as far as this type of injury is concerned is the chest X-ray (CXR). This will show up rib fractures, a pneumothorax, or a haemothorax and possibly injuries to the major blood vessels.

An ECG will be abnormal if there has been damage to the heart, and a check on the haemoglobin level is useful to make some estimate of the blood loss.

Chapter 20

Wounds and bleeding

Wounds to the skin and/or the underlying soft tissues, e.g., subcutaneous fat/muscle, etc, may be of two main types:

(1) Open, where there is a break in the skin or mucous membrane which allows blood to escape and infective organisms, e.g., bacteria, to enter.
(2) Closed, where there is bleeding under the skin, which in time becomes apparent as bruising. Though blood is not 'spilt' it is still lost to the circulation, i.e., it is internal bleeding.

Classification of wounds

Contused

This is the classic injury caused by a blunt instrument, e.g., a hammer. The wound may be closed with just swelling or bruising in the area, or open where the skin has split, often in several directions. Where a highly vascular organ, e.g., spleen or liver underlies the bruise, there can be damage to this structure and extensive internal bleeding. Such wounds are much more difficult to suture than a straightforward incised wound and do not heal as well because of the areas of crushed dead tissue around the wound.

Lacerated

An open jagged wound such as would be caused by a sharp metal edge, e.g., a tin can, the skin and underlying tissue is torn and there is often a high risk of infection as the object producing the wound is frequently dirty.

Incised

This type of wound would be caused by a sharp knife or broken glass.

Puncture

These are usually small wounds but are a most worrying type as you have no way of knowing, when you are on site, the exact depth to which the weapon penetrated. They can be deceiving as there may be relatively little blood leaking out through the wound but there could be devastating internal bleeding if a highly vascular organ has been damaged.

Gun shot

Single bullet wound

These are caused by a projectile which may be of high or low velocity. The low velocity bullet will penetrate soft tissues damaging them and may smash bones or be deflected or stopped by them. A high velocity bullet tends to go straight through the patient with less deflection but causing immense damage due to the shock waves it produces, e.g., it can fracture a bone without actually touching it. They tend to leave small entry wounds and larger exit wounds.

Shot gun wounds

These tend to cause massive soft tissue damage especially when fired from close range. If fired from a longer distance, the patient tends to be 'peppered' with small wounds.

External haemorrhage

Invariably in any open wound many small capillaries are cut and these ooze blood persistently but not in great quantities. Occasionally however, a larger vessel is cut, e.g., a small artery or vein. Blood from a cut artery characteristically shoots out in spurts and is bright red in colour. When a vein is cut the blood loss is in a steady trickle and the blood is dark bluish-red in colour.

Treatment

Expose the wound and surrounding area in a good light, if necessary removing or cutting away damaged or contaminated clothing. If no foreign bodies are present, immediately apply direct pressure over the wound by placing a clean (preferably sterile) pad onto the wound and holding or bandaging it firmly into place. If there are foreign bodies present which can *easily* be removed do so. If however, they are deeply embedded apply pressure to both sides of the wound simultaneously in an attempt to slow down any haemorrhage, then pad the surrounding area and bandage in order to prevent movement of the embedded implement. Remember to keep the area as clean as possible, removing contaminated clothing and anything of a constricting nature, e.g., rings and watches. Examine the patient for underlying fractures and if none are found, lie the patient down and elevate the injured area, keeping the patient calm and quiet, comfortable and reassured.

Sterile dressings

These should be of a size large enough to cover the wound. If no foreign bodies or fractures are present, press the pad firmly down onto the wound making sure you do not touch the sterile parts of the dressing. It should be secured firmly in place with a bandage ensuring that the dressing is completely covered, if foreign bodies are present or the end of a bone is protruding use two or more dressings, the sterile part applied to the wound and folded back, serving as a bridge, taking pressure off the foreign body or the bone end. When secured in place with a bandage this should control the haemorrhage. Splinting may be necessary and pneumatic splints are ideal for the purpose as you provide both support and pressure.

Remember

(1) To check the pulse at regular intervals.
(2) To make sure the bleeding is controlled.
(3) To check the patient's other vital signs to determine if his condition is deteriorating or improving.
(4) To note down your findings and pass them on.

Do not

(1) Use a tourniquet. A pressure point may have to be used, i.e., the brachial or femoral.
(2) Cover the area with blankets so that the bleeding cannot be easily checked.

Internal haemorrhage

Internal haemorrhage means internal bleeding into one of the body cavities or into muscles or internal organs. For instance, a kick to the chest may fracture a rib which tears a blood vessel in the lung, bleeding then takes place into this organ. Internal bleeding may not be visible immediately, however, it may subsequently become apparent when the patient vomits up blood from an internal haemorrhage into his stomach for instance. Thus bleeding into the lungs may be coughed up as bloody sputum (an haemoptysis). Bleeding from a damaged kidney may become apparent as blood mixed with the urine (haematuria), whilst bleeding into the gut from a gastric ulcer may be vomited up (haematemesis).

It is possible however, that internal bleeding may never become evident, for instance a blow to the abdomen which results in a small laceration to the liver can result in bleeding into the abdominal cavity which, if it stops spontaneously, will remain unnoticed. However, should bleeding continue, the blood loss will soon become sufficient to drop the blood pressure and the patient will become shocked and quite possibly die if surgical intervention is not undertaken.

The effect of blood loss

Up to 10 per cent of a normal healthy person's blood volume may be lost with few, if any, physical signs detectable. However, as the amount of blood loss increases towards 20 per cent the patient's pulse rate increases and by the time that the loss has reached a third of the patient's blood volume he will start to shut down his peripheral circulation with the result that his extremeties become cold and grey. This is done in an attempt to maintain his blood pressure which may remain at relatively normal levels. With blood loss greater than 30 per cent, the patient's condition will deteriorate rapidly as he becomes shocked.

Amputations

In recent years advances in surgery have meant that amputated limbs or fingers can, in certain cases, be successfully reattached. In order that the patient has the best possible chance of successful surgery it is important that he and the severed part be delivered in as good a condition as possible. Too often severed fingers, hands or feet have been left at the scene or poorly treated so that surgery is unsuccessful. Here are some guidelines as to the management of cases of amputation.

(1) Notify the Accident and Emergency Department of the Hospital concerned as soon as possible giving them an estimated time of arrival.

(2) Render all necessary treatment to the patient.

(3) If necessary reposition the partially amputated part by gentle manipulation and maintain the position by a loose well padded dressing and splint.

(4) Where a limb has been fully amputated control the haemorrhage by sterile dressings, pressure and elevation and if this does not control the bleeding, use the relevant pressure point.

(5) Preserve the amputated parts by sealing in a plastic bag which should be padded and placed in a container with ice. The ice should not come into direct contact with the amputated part, nor should you use dry ice or any other preservative fluids.

(6) Do not waste time cleaning the amputated part, it is unnecessary. Detergents may damage the tissue. Any cleaning will be carried out at the hospital.

(7) Transport the patient to the hospital as quickly as possible.

(8) Do not assure the patient that reattachment will be possible.

Chapter 21

Thermal injuries

Burns and scalds

Thermal injuries include burns of all types (i.e., extreme heat, chemical, electrical, radiation, etc), and scalds from both boiling liquids and steam. All of these different types of phenomena initially damage the skin and subsequently the underlying tissue, and thus we classify burns as either:

(1) Superficial (first and second degree, or partial thickness).
(2) Deep (third degree or full thickness).

Superficial burns

These only involve the topmost layers of the skin (*see Figure 21.1*) and first degree burns are characterized by redness (erythema) and pain. A second degree burn, which is slightly deeper, produces some swelling and blistering as well as the pain and erythema. Superficial burns tend to heal well within a week or two, with little if any residual scarring.

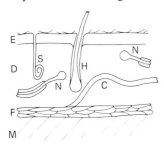

Figure 21.1 Section through normal skin: E = Epidermis, covered with dead cells; D = Dermis; S = Sweat gland; N = Nerve ending; H = Hair follicle; C = Capillary; F = Subcutaneous Fat; M = Muscle.

Deep burns

These involve the full thickness of the skin and sometimes underlying structures, e.g., fat and muscle. The specialized structures such as the sweat glands, hair follicles and nerve endings which lie within the dermis are also destroyed and do not regenerate. A deep burn usually takes a considerable time to heal, e.g., months rather than weeks, and frequently skingrafting is required. Even with these highly sophisticated techniques scarring is considerable.

Estimating the extent of the burns

When a burn patient is admitted some estimate has to be made of the extent of the body surface which is damaged. This is done by using a chart (*see Figure 21.2*) in which the body has been divided up into sections, e.g., arm, leg and trunk, and the surface area of each section is expressed as a percentage of the total area of the whole body.

By estimating the percentage of burned skin and deciding whether this is partial or full thickness, some idea can be obtained as to the prognosis for the patient and also his likely requirements as far as fluid replacement is concerned.

Complications of burns

Respiratory damage

Many substances, e.g., certain upholstery materials when ignited produce noxious fumes which can cause problems if inhaled. Further, the inhalation of hot air, fumes or steam can give rise to burns of the air passages which can indeed be fatal. These facts should always be borne in mind when attending to anyone who has been involved in a fire, particularly where there are burns to the head and neck.

Infection

The raw area of a burn is kept moist by body fluids which constantly 'weep out' from beneath the damaged skin. This moist area is a perfect breeding ground for bacteria, and burns, if contaminated, very rapidly become severely infected. Infected burns are difficult to treat, and are frequently the cause of death in a severely burned patient.

Fluid loss

The constant oozing of body fluids described in the previous para-

S&N CHART FOR ESTIMATING SEVERITY OF BURN WOUND

NAME_____WARD_____ NUMBER_____DATE____
AGE_____   ADMISSION WEIGHT_____

LUND AND BROWDER CHARTS

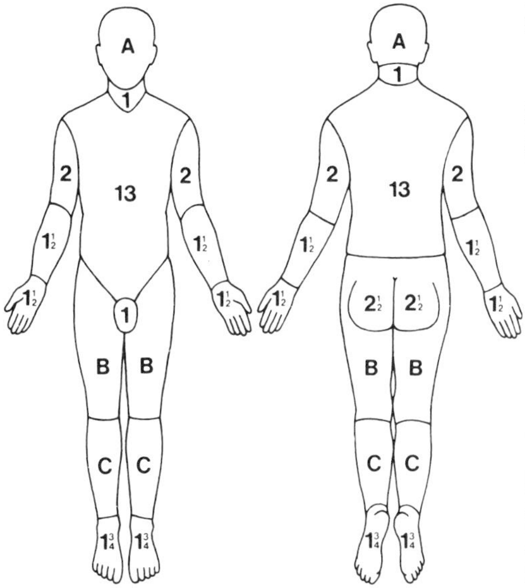

IGNORE
SIMPLE ERYTHEMA

Partial thickness loss
(PTL)
Full thickness loss
(FTL)

REGION	% PTL	FTL
HEAD		
NECK		
ANT. TRUNK		
POST. TRUNK		
RIGHT ARM		
LEFT ARM		
BUTTOCKS		
GENITALIA		
RIGHT LEG		
LEFT LEG		
TOTAL BURN		

RELATIVE PERCENTAGE OF BODY SURFACE AREA
AFFECTED BY GROWTH

AREA	AGE 0	1	5	10	15	ADULT
A = ½ OF HEAD	9½	8½	6½	5½	4½	3½
B = ½ OF ONE THIGH	2¾	3¼	4	4½	4½	4¾
C = ½ OF ONE LEG	2½	2½	2¾	3	3¼	3½

Figure 21.2 Chart for estimating the extent of burns. Reproduced by
kind permission of Smith and Nephew Pharmaceuticals Limited.

graph can, if the burned area is considerable, lead a highly significant loss of fluid and if this is not replaced rapidly the patient can
become shocked and die. Replacing fluid is an urgent priority in a
case where a significant percentage of the body surface has been
burned.

Treatment of burns

Initially remove yourself and the patient from the danger area, make sure his airway is open and check his breathing.

Where the head and face are involved, leave the burned area exposed and if the patient is unconscious insert an airway and monitor his breathing carefully.

If there are burns to the neck, an icepack or cold compresses may be applied to the area and if the patient is conscious he may be given some ice to suck. Where you are dealing with an unconscious patient an airway and close monitoring of his breathing may be needed.

Where other parts of the body are involved, such as the torso and limbs, the burns should be covered with a burns sheet, or freshly laundered cotton sheet or pillow case. If you arrive within 15 minutes of the incident occurring, superficial burns may be cooled using cold water. Anything of a constrictive nature, e.g., rings, watches, bracelets, etc. should be quickly removed, remembering that it is often easier to remove a ring with the hand immersed in cold water.

Burned clothing should not be removed as it has been sterilized by the heat, however if the clothing is soaked with hot water it should be carefully removed immediately.

Please remember not to apply any home-spun remedies to the burns such as butter, ointments, etc., as these will only contaminate the wound.

If blisters are appearing, do not rupture them. If the burns cover a significant percentage of the body area, the patient will need an intravenous infusion started and analgesics for the pain. Oxygen may well be required, particularly where there is an indication that the respiratory tract may have been involved.

Chemical burns

Remember not to be contaminated yourself when attending at an incident of this type.

Flood the area involved with running water under low pressure making sure that the water can drain away safely, then when the flushing is well under way remove the contaminated clothing carefully. You should continue drenching the area until all the chemical has been removed.

The burned area should be covered with a clean, preferably sterile, dressing or burns sheet, as for a burn caused by dry heat and the patient admitted making sure he is accompanied by all the necessary information, e.g., what type of chemical is involved.

Electrical burns

Electrical burns are all considered to be deep as the current surges through the tissue damaging all the structures in its path. There is an entry point at the area of contact and an exit point where the body has 'earthed'. Though the contact points may appear small, the underlying damage is often great.

Do remember that before you approach a patient who has been electrocuted, you should make sure that he is not still in contact with the source.

Patients who have been electrocuted may have other injuries such as fractures, dislocations or torn muscles. However, the most important problem is that they may have suffered a cardiac arrest. Having ensured that they are no longer in contact with the electrical source, check their breathing and pulse with a view to starting CPR should these be absent.

Having examined the casualty carefully and noted exit and entrance wounds, dress the wounds with dry sterile dressings and transport urgently to hospital.

Burns to special areas

Eyes

Burns to the eyes are especially important as damage to the cornea can lead to scarring and blindness. Whenever you are dealing with injuries to this area ensure that the eyes are copiously flushed with cool water under low pressure, not forgetting to evert both lids. When you are sure that the eyes are cooled, apply a damp sterile dressing over the injured eye and a dry dressing over the uninjured eye to minimize eye movement. Do not forget to keep the patient fully informed as to why you are doing this.

Mouth and throat

Any area of tissue which has been burned swells. This does not matter if the burn is on the back of the arm, but where the airway is involved as with the mouth and throat, close monitoring of the patient's breathing is mandatory, as these tissues can swell very rapidly and obstruct the airway.

Hypothermia

The normal body temperature lies between 36 and 37 degrees C, hypothermia is said to exist when the temperature is below this. If the temperature is 34 degrees C and upwards, the hypothermia is said to be mild, where the temperature lies between 32–34 degrees C it is moderate and if the patient's temperature is 31 degrees C or less the hypothermia is severe.

The normal temperature is maintained by the circulation of blood and there is a controlling mechanism situated in the part of the brain called the hypothalamus which acts as a thermostat.

There are four groups of people who are peculiarly prone to hypothermia, they are:

(1) Babies
(2) The sick
(3) The elderly
(4) Derelicts and alcoholics

There is a certain amount of overlap between groups (2) and (3) as some elderly people will also be invalids.

Babies and very small children are prone to hypothermia as the 'thermostat' in their hypothalamus is not fully developed at birth and hence does not adjust their body temperature as well as that of an older child. Sick people, particularly those for instance with a stroke, tend to be unable to move around to keep their temperature up whilst others may have disorders such as myxoedema (see page 123), under which circumstances they are particularly prone to hypothermia. Elderly patients are also prone to hypothermia, not only because of illness but because they are less energetic and thus move around less than a younger person and also they are likely to be less well off financially and many will be unable to afford adequate heating and clothing for the cold winter months. Furthermore because of the financial aspect and other factors such as a poor appetite their diet may leave much to be desired. Finally, alcoholics and derelicts often have no adequate housing and because of this can often lie for prolonged periods in a drunken stupor under conditions which make hypothermia a likely occurrence. Also alcohol tends to dilate blood vessels and increase the rate of heat loss thus precipitating hypothermia.

Clinical features of hypothermia

In the initial stages of hypothermia the patient begins to feel cold and shiver, he gradually slows down both physically and mentally, and his skin feels cold to the touch. Gradually as the temperature falls, his extremities become blue or white, his respiration rate slows, and his breathing is shallow. The pulse rate also slows and the pulse itself becomes barely palpable even in a large artery such as the femoral. Then his level of consciousness changes as he becomes drowsy, stuporose, comatose and finally death ensues.

Treatment

(1) Protect the airway.
(2) Support respiration as necessary.
(3) Prevent further reduction of body temperature.
(4) Commence passive rewarming of the patient. Do not actively heat the patient with electric fires or similar, as too rapid rewarming can be dangerous.

Remember to remove clothing if it is wet and not to move the patient unnecessarily. If the patient is fully conscious he may be given warm, sweet drinks but never *alcohol*. Until he reaches hospital the patient's rewarming should be purely passive with him being wrapped in a thermal blanket with the shiny side inwards. He can then be covered with conventional blankets. Great care needs to be taken with rewarming of an elderly patient as they can become shocked or a fatal arrhythmia may be induced.

The thermal blanket

This is a thin, aluminium foil sheet which sometimes has a plastic backing, which folds up to a relatively small size and is extremely light. Its main use is to reduce the amount of heat lost through the body by radiation and it also acts as a conductor of heat when used in conjunction with conventional blankets for continued insulation.

Method of use   The patient is removed to a waterproof and windproof shelter and completely cocooned in a thermal blanket with the shiny side nearest the body, the head being included but being careful not to obstruct the airway. Conventional blankets if they are available are then wrapped around the thermal blanket and the patient is then kept out of the wet and cold. If the patient is conscious remove wet clothing and dry the patient, applying the thermal blanket next to the skin. If he is unconscious, do not trouble to remove the wet clothing but apply the thermal blanket over it.

Exposure

This is a condition which is, with the application of common sense, is very often avoidable. The patient gets cold in bad climatic conditions, therefore he is wet and exhausted.

At first he slows down physically and intellectually, losing coordination, becoming confused, perhaps aggressive and shivering violently. There is then a gradual deterioration in his level of consciousness until he becomes comatose and subsequently dies. Initially he should be rested and sheltered from the elements and kept warm with minimal handling. If he is conscious, warm sweet drinks are permissible and immediate transfer to hospital where passive rewarming will be continued or under some circumstances active rewarming in a water bath, or using radiant heat may be considered.

Frostbite

Frostbite occurs where there is actual freezing of exposed extremities such as fingers, or the tip of the nose. Where a finger is involved it will for instance become cold, white, numb and stiff with gangrene occurring later.

The treatment is to safeguard the patient's general condition to remove any restrictions from the area, such as rings, and then to rewarm the extremity passively. Do not ever use active rewarming techniques or rub or slap the affected area.

Heat exhaustion

This is due to the excessive loss of salt and water when a patient perspires copiously. The patient becomes exhausted, has muscle cramps and eventually the skin becomes cold, pale and moist and when the pulse is taken it is noted to be weak and rapid. Often the patient's temperature is normal or only slightly raised.

The immediate treatment is to rest the patient in the coolest available environment and to administer sips of cool, slightly salted water prior to transfer to hospital.

Heat stroke

This is most frequently found in new arrivals to tropical climates, particularly where there is a high relative humidity. The patient's temperature is raised and the skin is hot and dry. There is little or no perspiration and the pulse is strong and easily felt at the wrist.

Gradually as his condition deteriorates he may become delirious and finally lapse into coma.

The treatment is to reduce the temperature rapidly by tepid sponging, fanning or if necessary immersing in a cold bath. Antipyretics such as aspirin may be administered and the patient hospitalized urgently.

Chapter 22

Infectious diseases

In spite of all the modern advances in medical treatment, and the widespread availability of antibiotics in particular, infectious diseases are still a major cause for concern. A further complication is that modern travel methods mean that diseases can be spread rapidly and may bring people into contact with many exotic tropical infections. Some of these diseases can be extremely dangerous for a patient and occasionally the community also. Infectious diseases are caused by the invasion of the human body by another type of organism. These can range in size from a submicroscopic virus to a 6 metre, (20 foot) long tapeworm.

The main classes of organisms

Viruses

These are very small, they live and reproduce inside other cells, and usually can only be visualized by the use of an electron microscope.

Bacteria

These are very small but they can be seen with a light microscope. They may live inside other organisms or in a free state.

Protozoa

These are similar in size to a red blood cell.

Helminths (worms)

These range in size from the microscopic to those which may be 6 metres, (20 foot) long.

Insects

These are usually visible to the naked eye.

Fungi

These inhabit the skin and mucous membranes or may enter the body.
There are literally thousands of different types of invading organisms which can vary enormously in their effects and hence in the diseases which they cause

Diseases caused by invading organisms

Viruses

The common cold, influenza, measles, mumps, chicken pox, hepatitis, herpes, polio, small pox, etc. There is usually no specific cure for these diseases and they may vary widely in severity, some lasting only a few days and curing themselves, the patient having no further problems whilst others can leave a patient permanently crippled. Some may remain dormant in the body for many years and do not manifest themselves until the patient is weakened by another disease.

Bacteria

These are classified accordingly to their shape, e.g., Cocci are round, Bacilli are rod-shaped, Spirilla are spiral shaped, and then by the family to which they belong. Each bacterium causes a specific disease, e.g., *Mycobacterium tuberculosis* causes tuberculosis, *Mycobacterium leprae* causes leprosy. Other important diseases caused by bacteria include dysentery, food poisoning, meningitis, several forms of venereal disease, typhoid, cholera, pneumonia, whooping cough and hundreds more.

Protozoa

Malaria, amoebiasis and many other tropical diseases. Trichomonas is a common genito-urinary disease in the United Kingdom which is caused by protozoa.

Helminths

Tapeworms, round-worms, thread-worms and many tropical forms including Bilharzia.

Insects

Scabies, lice, fleas.

Fungi

Thrush, athlete's foot, ringworm.

Spread of infection

In order for a disease to spread, the organism has to get from one host (individual) to another, these are the common methods they use.

Droplet

Bacteria or viruses may be coughed out into the air in tiny droplets and then inhaled by another person, as occurs for instance in tuberculosis and measles.

Infected objects

Infected articles of clothing, cooking and domestic items, infected dressings and syringes, sputum, faeces, etc, e.g., hepatitis.

Direct touch

Kissing, sexual intercourse, unhygienic nursing techniques, e.g., glandular fever, gonorrhoea.

Penetration of the skin

Wounds, insect bites, etc, e.g., tetanus caused by an infection entering via a small wound, whilst malaria occurs following an insect bite.

Ingestion

This may be food or drink or objects which are put into the mouth, e.g., dysentery, tapeworm and food poisoning.

Carriers

In order to survive some organisms have to exist in carriers.

Human carriers

A carrier may have the actual disease or occasionally may have no symptoms whatsoever and thus be much more dangerous because neither they or anyone else realize that they are infecting other people. A carrier may be infectious before he becomes symptomatic and hence they are unaware that they have the disease and are spreading it (e.g., whooping cough, measles, etc), or for a long time after they have recovered (e.g., cholera, typhoid), or even without having obviously been infected at all.

Animal carriers

Some diseases may exist naturally in animals but are capable of infecting man as well, e.g., rabies (dogs), brucellosis (cows), anthrax (animal hides).

Other diseases use a vector to carry them from one person to another and in some cases to complete their life cycle, e.g., flies infecting food, mosquitoes carrying malaria or yellow fever.

How the spread can be prevented

Rapid notification

All medical and paramedical staff must be on the alert for these diseases. At the slightest suspicion a report should be made to the Community Health Physician.

Isolation

The infected person may have to be isolated from other susceptible people. Any person who *might* have been infected with certain diseases may also have to be isolated. Isolation may have to be for several days or weeks (quarantine). In some diseases this is compulsory.

Disinfection

All infected articles must be sterilized or in some cases destroyed.

Immunization

By immunizing an individual we make them immune from, or less susceptible to the infection. Some diseases like measles give a complete immunity after cure, others like gonorrhoea do not. Examples of immunization include BCG for tuberculosis, measles vaccination.

Strict attention to the rules of hygiene

This is mandatory for all health care personnel, masks and gowns should be worn and you should wash between attending patients. Particular care has to be taken in kitchens and by food handlers, etc.

Tracing and removing the source of infection where possible

This is not always easy but is important in order to prevent further out-breaks of the disease.

General management of infectious diseases

In order to contain infection in the patient and prevent infection by airborne droplets, you should wear a mask and indeed the patient himself may be supplied with a mask.

Wear protective clothing as is provided (gowns, hats, gloves).
Scrub your hands and nails thoroughly.
Brush your hair and clothing and hang the clothing so that it is exposed to the light and air.
Shower or bath as soon as possible.
Make sure that your inoculations are kept up to date.
Do not handle the patient more than is absolutely necessary.
Disinfect your vehicle with the recommended chemical.
Do not handle dressings, blood, sputum, faeces, urine, etc without gloves.

Some useful terms

Endemic

The constant level of disease prevalence in an area.

Epidemic

Any rise from the normal level, e.g., one case of smallpox would be an epidemic, but many cases of influenza would be needed before it is termed epidemic. Epidemics can be sudden and explosive, e.g.,

50 cases of food poisoning occurring in 24 hours, or may be seasonal, e.g., epidemics in every spring or summer.

Pandemic

Epidemic of worldwide proportions, e.g., historical episodes of plague and cholera.

Sporadic

Unconnected cases occurring at various times.

Incubation

Diseases may be said to have started when the organism has entered the body, but symptoms only appear after a variable length of time, this is the incubation period, and the patient may be infectious during this time.

Chapter 23

Major incidents

Major incidents are fortunately not frequent occurrences, but when they happen they will cause panic amongst the people involved and stress on the emergency services which have to deal with them. Major incidents or major disasters are defined as any incident, which because of the number of casualties, requires special arrangements to deal with it, rather than the normal emergency procedures. The type of incident can vary (air crashes, terrorist incidents, mining disasters, etc), each bringing its own particular problems.

The senior police officer at the site will be in over-all charge of any major incident, and he will co-ordinate the operation with the help of senior officers from the other services, with the main objective always being the preservation of life.

The natural reaction of someone attending at the scene of a major incident, is to rush in and try to render aid to the injured, this, if you are alone and in a mass casualty situation, is going to be of little help. The most important thing is to alert the emergency services as every Health Authority has a Major Incident plan formulated which must be put into action in order that the best utilization of trained personnel, vehicles and resources is made, and priority casualties can be treated and transported to hospital without delay.

Duty of the ambulance service in a major incident

In any mass casualty situation organization and planning is of the utmost importance, it is the duty of the Ambulance Service to:

(1) Arrange for there to be sufficient ambulances and first-aid equipment readily available to ensure the preservation of life, the treatment and the transportation of the injured to medical centres.
(2) Alert and organize medical and paramedical teams and first-aid organizations.

(3) To co-ordinate medical arrangements at the scene, with the Site Medical Officer and the designated hospitals through the Liaison Officer as the situation requires.
(4) To ensure, after the early concentration of ambulances, a steady flow of vehicles at the scene to transport the injured.

The duty of the first ambulance at the scene therefore, should be to give a precise, accurate and immediate report to his control.

Driver – to stay with vehicle

(1) Confirm the exact location of the incident.
(2) Describe the best access and egress routes.
(3) A description of the incident as it can be seen from the vehicle.
(4) What other services are in attendance or required.
(5) Log all messages and wait the arrival of the Incident Officer.
(6) Park adjacent to the Police Control Point with blue flashing emergency lights on in order to identify the vehicle as the temporary incident control post.

Attendant – to carry out a brief reconnaissance

The situation report should cover the following:

(1) Confirmation that this is a Major Incident.
(2) An estimate of the number of casualties.
(3) A description of any additional hazards.
(4) Contact Police and Fire Officers and in consultation with them set up the following:
    (a) An Ambulance Incident Control Point
    (b) An ambulance parking area
    (c) An ambulance loading point
    (d) A first-aid equipment point
    (e) A casualty clearing site
    (f) A stretcher bearers' assembly point
    (g) The site for a temporary mortuary (manned by a Police Officer)

As further ambulances arrive they should be parked in the designated area and the drivers must stay with their vehicles, blue flashing emergency lights being turned off. The attendants must report to the Incident Control Point and the Incident Officer.

All Ambulance Officers are to report to the Incident Control Point and the Incident Officer.

All the aforementioned points should be covered by a Marshal to co-ordinate the smooth running of the service.

All voluntary first-aiders should report to the Ambulance Incident Officer.

Specific areas

First-aid point

This is where supplies of equipment are kept for issue to the services dealing with casualties.

Stretcher bearers' assembly point

This is a designated location where volunteer stretcher bearers can be organized.

Casualty clearing point

This, where possible, should be provided with shelter and should be sited on firm ground. The Site Medical Officer will be in charge, and his main objective is the sorting of Casualties into priority groups.

Ambulance loading point

This should be adjacent to the Casualty Clearing area and again needs firm ground and turning space for ambulances.

Ambulance parking point

Here, additional ambulances are parked, with the driver inside and ready to proceed to the Loading Point as and when they are required. They should not cause obstruction at the scene.

Ambulance incident control point

This should be situated in an area where all three emergency services can be adjacent for good communication and liaison.

Mortuary

This should be sited near the Casualty Clearing Area, but preferably out of sight. It will be manned by the Police.

Bomb alerts

Incidents involving bombs are increasingly becoming a factor of everyday life. Ambulance crews on receipt of such a call should proceed discreetly, without using blue lights and two-tone horns, to a stand-by point which will be specified, and which will be approximately half a mile from the reported location.

(1) Do not approach these incidents until the Police give permission.
(2) The radio-telephone should not be used as experience has proven that such transmissions can trigger the device.
(3) Do not move bodies or items of luggage, shopping bags, etc.
(4) Temporary facilities such as Contact Points, Loading Points, Casualty Clearing Stations, etc., should be at least two hundred yards further back than is normal.

Casualties

Particular attention should be paid to the assessment of the patient's condition and the observation of any changes. Due to the dramatic effect of the incident a patient may be confused and unaware of the extent of his injuries. The management of the patient with multiple injuries will require great skill and the use of many different techniques in carrying out the appropriate treatment. Ensure at all times the safety of yourself and the patient.

Possible injuries in a major incident

Burns

(1) Burns covering large areas which can produce shock.
(2) Facial burns and the inhalation of fumes can cause airway problems.
(3) Burns may be complicated by fractures and other injuries.

Chest injuries

(1) Failure of the mechanism of respiration due to the rib-cage being fractured in several places so that the chest wall loses its rigidity (flail chest).
(2) Pneumothorax.
(3) Haemothorax.
(4) Direct damage to the lungs and pleura.

Severe haemorrhage

Severe bleeding both internal and external and from fractures. The size of the wound may give you little indication of the severity. You will have no idea of the depth, and direction of penetration, which may involve large blood vessels and major organs. Open wounds may be complicated by embedded foreign bodies such as glass, rubble or missiles. The signs of shock due to blood loss may be the only indication of the severity of internal bleeding.

Abdominal injuries

Protrusion of organs with a high risk of contamination of the peritoneal cavity.

Head injuries

Concussion or compression may occur and there may be compound fractures with contamination of the meninges. Ringing in the ears and temporary or permanent deafness may hinder your assessment of the patient.

Multiple fractures

Many casualties may suffer more than one fracture. There may also be crush injuries and the limb may be fractured in more than one place.

Amputation

Amputated or partly amputated limbs are common.

Crush injuries

Casualties may be buried under rubble for long periods of time.

Hysteria

People separated from family and friends panic.

Transportation of dangerous substances

With the increasing use of toxic and radio-active substances by the industries of the Developed World, transportation of these chemicals is commonplace and incidents related to their spillage or leakage are frequent.

Problems may be caused by a substance exploding, whilst others will ignite spontaneously on exposure to air. Some volatilize when not under pressure and as gases or vapours asphyxiate bystanders, whilst others burn, or poison those involved in various ways. When called to an incident of this nature remember *danger*.

Do not rush in.
Assess the situation.
No smoking.
Get assistance and advice.
Estimate damage and casualties.
Remember your own safety.

The driver may have been trained in what to do if involved in an accident, always ask his advice initially. Do remember that when you are attending such an incident your initial action should be one of passing as much information to your control as you can possibly obtain by viewing from a safe distance. The situation report should include:

(1) (a) Confirmation of the location
    (b) The nature of the incident
    (c) Name of the vehicle owner
    (d) Vehicle registration number
    (e) Vehicle fleet number
    (f) Any leakage visible and where from.
(2) All the information displayed on the UKHIS label or Kemler Code. (*See Figure 23.1*)
    (a) Hazchem number
    (b) Type of hazard warning diamond (*see Figure 23.2*)
    (c) Substance identification number and name if displayed
    (d) Emergency telephone number if displayed.
(3) Whether Police or Fire Service are in attendance.
(4) Number of casualties and whether trapped, is the driver injured or contaminated in any way.
(5) Go to the scene (if it is safe to do so) make a quick reconnaissance and check on the accuracy of your initial information).
(6) Keep as far as possible 'up wind' of the vapour and 'up hill' on any spillage. Take care not to get splashed or walk in the spillage.
(7) Wear protective gloves and do not touch or smell any substance.

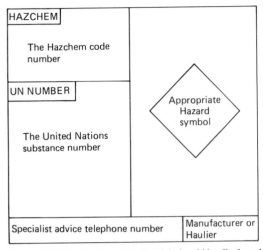

Figure 23.1 The Hazchem label which should be displayed on the rear and both sides of the vehicle. It has an orange background with black lettering.

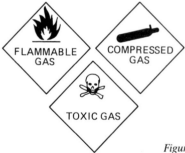

Figure 23.2 Some examples of hazard symbols.

(8) Do not engage in rescue work, personal safety is paramount, wait until the incident is declared safe by the Fire Officer.

(9) Do not use radio or any form of electrical equipment in the vicinity of the incident as this can be a source of ignition.

(10) Do not allow smoking in the area.

(11) Treat priorities in the normal way when attending to the patient.

Hazchem labels

The majority of tankers carrying dangerous substances display the *Hazchem* label, which has an orange background with black lettering and should be displayed on the rear and both sides of the vehicle (*see Figure 23.1*).

Chapter 24

Emergency childbirth

Ambulance personnel will only rarely be required to assist in a delivery, as the majority of patients receive antenatal care and are able to summon aid early in labour. The patients who may present as emergencies are:

(1) Those patients who have not sought antenatal care.
(2) Patients who have a very short labour.
(3) Those who for various reasons, (e.g., teenage pregnancies in the unmarried) have tried to hide their pregnancy.

Any person who is concerned with caring for a woman in labour should ensure that there is *minimum* interference, it should be remembered that the patient may have had a previous confinement, and is to some extent able to assess the stage of labour she has reached, and therefore her comments should not be ignored. Attendants must stay calm, childbirth is a natural process and should proceed uneventfully so reassure the parents.

Normal labour

First stage

This is the longest stage and prepares the birth canal to permit the safe passage of the baby. In a prima gravida (i.e., a patient having her first baby) it can last for up to 18 hours but is generally shorter with second and subsequent confinements. The first stage of labour starts with a 'show', a plug of mucus either white or reddish-brown which comes away from the cervix. The membrane may rupture (breaking of the waters). The baby is surrounded by 2–3 pints of watery amniotic fluid, and at any time during labour this fluid can escape in a trickle or a gush. Contractions of the uterus occur, which usually start in the lower back and radiate around to the bottom of the abdomen, the contractions increase in frequency from perhaps one every 30 minutes up to one every 2–3 minutes and are, generally speaking, uncomfortable to painful. They open up the cervix until it is wide enough to allow the baby to pass. As a general rule the more frequent and stronger the contractions are, the more advanced is the labour.

Second stage

This is the actual birth of the baby, and the mother feels she wants to 'push' or may feel a sensation of wanting to open her bowels, as gradually the top of the baby's head becomes visible. This stage can last for up to half-an-hour in a prima gravida or as short a time as a couple of minutes in the second and subsequent pregnancies. As the woman pushes or 'bears down' the baby is pushed along the birth canal, eventually stretching the vaginal orifice. Sometimes a tear occurs but this is later repaired by suturing. Usually the baby's head is born first followed by his shoulders, arms, body and legs. At this stage he is still attached to the placenta by the umbilical cord.

Third stage

The placenta, or after-birth, has to separate from the wall of the uterus and the blood vessels in that structure contract in order to prevent haemorrhage. When the placenta has completely separated (up to 20 minutes after birth) it is expelled down the birth canal.

Management

(1) In the first stage of labour ambulance personnel should move the patient from home to hospital in the normal manner. She can sit up or lie down which ever she prefers and may be offered Entonox. If her membranes have ruptured she must be transported lying down.

(2) (a) If the patient shows signs of the second stage she should not be moved from home.

  (b) Notify your control immediately of the ambulance location and request them to summon assistance from the Community Midwife and a general practitioner.

  (c) If in transit continue on to hospital unless the birth is imminent, in which case the ambulance should be parked in a quiet safe place until delivery is completed.

  (d) Remove your jacket and roll up your sleeves.

  (e) Reassure the mother and ask her to undress, preferably having the husband or a female relative with you.

(f) Check that the bed or stretcher is adequate and allow the mother to lie on her back supported by two or three pillows. Cover her with two blankets, one for the upper part and one for the lower, keeping her warm and avoiding undue exposure.

(g) Wash your hands if possible and open your maternity pack.

(h) As the head is being born do not touch it but ask the mother to pant with her contractions. This gives a more controlled delivery and can minimize damage to mother and baby.

(i) Once the head has emerged there is usually a short pause and at this time check that the umbilical cord is not around the baby's neck, if it is, ask the mother not to push and carefully slide the cord over the baby's head.

(j) The cord will only rarely be tight enough to necessitate clamping and cutting, if this is necessary however, use the two clamps in your delivery pack, placing them about two inches apart on the cord. Make sure they are tightly closed and then cut between the clamps unwinding the cord from around the baby's neck.

(k) Following the head, the shoulders and body will then be born. The attendant should hold the baby firmly by the shoulders remembering that it is wet and slippery. Guide him upwards towards the mother's abdomen. Do not pull on the cord.

(l) The infant should cry immediately. Lie the baby on its side to allow any fluid to drain out of the nose and mouth. Clear his nose and mouth gently with the mucus extractor. The mucus extractor only needs to be inserted ¼- inch into the nostrils and about ½-inch into the mouth. Wrap the infant in a dry, warm baby-wrap, covering his head but leaving his face exposed. Lie him on his mother's abdomen on his side. New-born babies are often blue at birth but become pink fairly quickly. Note the time and condition of the baby at birth.

(m) The cord should not be cut once the baby is born except by the midwife or doctor.

(n) Should the infant not breathe, mouth to mouth or nose resuscitation should be started with tiny puffs of air and continued until medical aid has arrived. Make sure the baby is kept warm.

Third stage

In the event of an ambulance delivery it is not necessary to remain stationary during the third stage. Notify control that you are moving on towards the hospital and request that a midwife meet you on arrival there. The attendant should remain with the mother and should watch the mother for signs of haemorrhage. Should the placenta be delivered during the journey leave it attached to the baby. Collect all stained articles and note the time of delivery. If you have delivered the child at home, the mother should not be moved until the midwife or doctor requests this. Until their arrival observe and reassure the patient.

Complications

Abortion or miscarriage

This means the loss of the products of conception before the twenty-eighth week. If bleeding is severe or if the patient begins to appear shocked she should not be moved from home. The Obstetric Flying Squad or Emergency Obstetric Unit should be summoned and also the general practitioner. Observe the patient's general condition and save all stained articles for later inspection.

Ante-partum haemorrhage

This is bleeding from the twenty-eighth week of pregnancy up until the baby is born. If you are summoned to such a case remember that the mother should *not* be moved however slight the bleeding may be. The Obstetric Flying Squad or Emergency Obstetric Team must be summoned together with the general practitioner. If bleeding occurs during the journey ask ambulance control to have staff at the hospital entrance to assist you.

Eclampsia

Sometimes during the course of her pregnancy a mother may develop a rise in her blood pressure together with some swelling of the extremities (i.e., fingers, feet and ankles). Protein may be found in the urine and this condition is known as pre-eclampsia. If it is not detected and treated it may progress to full-blown eclampsia in which fits and/or coma occur. The immediate management of an eclamptic patient would be the same as that for an epileptic fit in which she is prevented from biting her tongue and injuring herself and when convulsions have ceased her airway is protected and she is kept in the three-quarters prone position. The patient must not be moved and the Obstetric Flying Squad should be summoned. If the patient has a fit in the ambulance, first-aid measures should be instituted as you are proceeding quickly to the maternity hospital.

Breech delivery

Rarely babies are born bottom (breech) first. It is essential that the attendant does not interfere too much with the delivery and allows the mother to deliver the baby by herself as far as possible. Do not encourage her to push, encourage her to pant.

Post-partum haemorrhage

Bleeding may occur at any time from immediately following the birth up to 6 weeks later. If the patient is still at home summon the Obstetric Flying Squad and observe her until they arrive. If you are in transit, proceed as quickly as possible to the nearest maternity unit. Whilst you are on your way the attendant can 'rub up' the uterus and thus encourage it to contract and control the bleeding. This is done by placing your hand on the mother's abdomen just below the umbilicus and massaging gently until you feel the uterus firm beneath your hand. Reassure the mother during this procedure.

Entonox

Entonox is an analgesic gas used for the relief of pain. It is an equal mixture of nitrous oxide and oxygen. The two gases are mixed together in one cylinder which may be recognized by its colour code (a blue cylinder with a white segmented neck), and the fact that it has a single pin index connection so that an Entonox cylinder will only fit an Entonox yoke. The portable Entonox unit is serviced by a D-size cylinder which when full contains 500 l of gas.

Entonox must be self-administered by the patient. There is no additive effect between Entonox and any other medication and it has little in the way of side-effects other than making the patient feel drowsy and light-headed. It helps to relieve pain and is effective for about 2 minutes after being stopped.

Use of the apparatus

(1) Entonox must be self-administered, therefore the patient must be conscious.
(2) The airway must always be clear.
(3) It is vital that a clear explanation and demonstration be given to the patient of what is required for it to work effectively.
(4) The use of a clear, closed mask of the correct size which establishes a good seal, is necessary.

(5) The cylinder must be fully opened, four good turns of the key.
(6) Allow the patient to inhale the gas for approximately 2 minutes in order to obtain maximum effect, or until the mask falls away if sooner. Monitor the patient carefully and check that the analgesic has taken effect.

You should never attempt to give Entonox to an unconscious patient, nor to one who has severe chest, head or facial injuries. Other groups of patients in which it is contra-indicated are drunks and drug addicts, elderly confused patients, violent patients, infants and those with the 'bends' (decompression disease).

Care of the apparatus

When changing the cylinder make sure that all the red plastic seal is removed otherwise leaks may occur. The cylinder should be turned on before fitting to the yoke as they sometimes jam, and the manoeuvre also clears any dust. If after fitting the cylinder correctly to the yoke it leaks at the connection, check the bulldog washer and turn or replace it as necessary. Clean the mask and tubing only with warm soapy water, but do not clean the yoke with water. If it has been exposed to exceptionally cold conditions, the gases will separate, shake the cylinder and listen for the sound of liquid as nitrous oxide will liquify at extreme temperatures. The cylinder should be immersed in warm water for 4–5 minutes and then inverted three times, gently shaking each time to help mix the gases.

Chapter 25
Patient handling

Two major causes of sickness absence in the ambulance service are gastro-intestinal problems and back pain. It is likely that the GI problems are related to the pressures of the job and the unsocial hours worked but the cause of the back pain is more complex. The obvious hazards would appear to be the handling and lifting of patients, but there are other contributing factors, for instance there are the effects of vibration on the spine during prolonged driving and the sudden changes from the relatively passive state work posture to the dynamic activity related to the manual movement of patients.

Research into the topic of back pain in the ambulance service is limited, but what evidence is available suggests that the handling of patients and equipment was the major cause. A further factor was the difficult conditions in which ambulancemen frequently have to operate, carrying heavy patients up and down staircases for instance.

The prevention of back pain has always been a problem and sickness absence statistics over the past decade indicate that the solutions tried so far have been unsuccessful in that the incidence of absence due to back pain has risen every year.

In the past, training in safe manual handling techniques was considered to be the ideal preventative measure. This concept is no longer accepted by those who specialize in manual handling research. A much broader approach is now recommended involving sickness absence and accident monitoring, the creation of safer systems at work, and finally suitable and supervized training.

If the hazards of moving patients manually are to be reduced and eventually eliminated, far greater consideration must be given to the systems of work in operation, including the equipment and vehicles used.

Safer patient handling

Basic assessment

(1) Before any patient is lifted or moved, they should be assessed with regard to their fundamental abilities and general condition. It is erroneous to consider ambulance personnel as specialized mobile porters. Recognition must be given to the fact that the ambulance crews are often the first members of the medical service to have contact with the patient and are thus often obliged to make primary medical decisions.

(2) Whenever possible patients should be encouraged to help move themselves within the limits of their capabilities, and they should be kept informed of what is likely to happen during any procedure.

(3) Maximum use should be made of any simple aids that may be available, sheets, blankets, towels and even a strong shirt or pyjama jacket can be utilized to reduce the stress of moving a heavy patient.

(4) Manual handling techniques should not be taught as a rigid drill, rather all staff should be encouraged to be competent and adaptable to the extent that they are able to select the appropriate lifts for the many and varying situations which may be encountered.

(5) It is not sufficient to provide students with a film and demonstration of lifting techniques. Lifting is a practical skill and as such, must be taught carefully and followed by properly supervized practice.

(6) For those involved in regular manual handling activities, refresher courses are essential in order to check current performance and also to introduce new ideas.

Principles of lifting

Without becoming involved in detailed anatomical, physiological and bio-mechanical principles, it is generally accepted that the human body functions most effectively as a lifting machine when:

(1) The spine is maintained in a correct natural posture.

(2) The spine is used as a link between the upper and lower limbs.

(3) The power of the legs is exploited in a variety of ways to provide the force needed to move the patient. The legs operate best when the knee and hip joints are used in mid-range.

(4) Maximum use is made of momentum and the forces that can be generated by the patient's own body.

(5) Smooth, natural, rhythmic techniques are far safer than jerky rigid movements.
(6) A good lift starts at the feet, and good foot position throughout the lift is vitally important.
(7) The load is kept as close to the lifter as possible and is best placed when held in contact with the body of the lifter.
(8) Loads are not to be moved the slightest bit further than is absolutely necessary.
(9) Lifting and carrying time is kept to an absolute minimum at all times.
(10) Lifters should always be aware of their limitations and not lift loads which feel too heavy. They should also seek assistance whenever necessary.
(11) Rest periods are a vital component of any lifting routine and must be taken in order to enable the spinal system to recover.

Lifting techniques

Because of the infinite and ever developing techniques of safe patient moving and handling, it is only possible to describe examples of some of the more recent introductions. As lifts using stretchers and other equipment have been covered in other sections, attention will be given to seated transfers.

Single operative manoeuvres

Momentum transfer

This is used to transfer patients from chair to chair, bed to chair, and chair to toilet or commode.

The patient is seated with knees and hips at a right angle (*see Figure 25.1*). His feet should be flat on the floor and sufficiently far apart to permit the lifter to place one foot between them. The other foot is placed in line with the object onto which the patient is being transferred.

The lifter's body is lowered by bending the hips and knees and then the patient is held by passing the hands under his axilla and holding him with a firm but gentle grasp over the upper back.

Momentum for the movement is initiated by gently rocking the patient, the transfer is made by gently swinging the patient across to the new position.

Points to note:

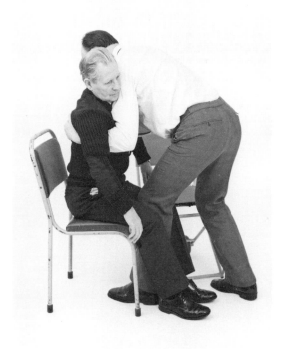

Figure 25.1 A patient being moved using momentum transfer.

(1) The patient should be encouraged to co-operate with the manoeuvre but not to be too eager.
(2) Normally three rocking motions are sufficient to ensure an easy transfer.
(3) Always swing the patient's weight from one foot to the other. Remember to maintain a steady controlled rhythm.

Double knee lock momentum transfer

This manoeuvre is for use primarily on patients who are unable to assist in their lift and/or have some form of increased muscle tone. The patient is seated with his hips and knees at right angles and feet together flat on the floor. The lifter positions himself in such a way that the patient's feet are held between his own, the patient's knees are then held firmly together by the lifter's knees. If this pressure causes discomfort, it is recommended that a folded towel be placed across the patient's knees to reduce the pressure.

Squatting down to achieve the correct height, the lifter holds the patient as in the previous lift, or makes use of a folded towel or ambulance sheet (*see Figure 25.2*).

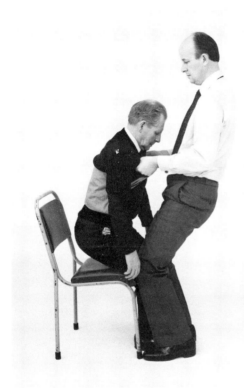

Figure 25.2 A patient being moved using the double-knee-lock momentum transfer, and making use of an ambulance sheet.

Movement of the patient is initiated by the lifter leaning back on his knees. Once the patient is raised the feet are pivoted whilst at the same time pressure is applied by the lifter's knee on the side away from the direction of motion. This swings the patient onto the new seat. The locking pressure of the knees must be maintained throughout the manoeuvre as this prevents the patient's knees giving way or shooting into a straightened position. Once the patient is secure adjust his position.

The Durston flyer

Modified from a lifting technique used by physiotherapists, this simple manoeuvre enables patients with moderate abilities to be transferred from one seated position into another with minimal effort.

The two seats must be positioned at 90 degrees to one another. Assuming that the patient has a weak side, as is typical with a hemiplegic, the following procedure is adopted:

(1) Place the patient's feet firmly on the floor, checking that the knees are together and bent at 90 degrees.
(2) The direction of the lift is always towards the stronger side.
(3) Block the patient's weaker foot and knee to prevent any slipping or movement during the actual transfer.
(4) The patient is asked to link his fingers together and stretch his arms forward and across the lifter's hip on the weaker side.
(5) The lifter after checking that both the patient's position and his own are satisfactory, places his hands over the patient's shoulders and rests them on the shoulder blades. Greater security is achieved if the middle finger of each hand is located into the patient's axilla.
(6) With a gentle forward motion the patient is transferred by means of gentle pressure from the lifter's legs on the weak side. Control and guidance is maintained by the hands and fingers.
(7) This manoeuvre requires some practice before proficiency is achieved. The simplicity and minimal pressure that is required to transfer the patient have caused confusion in lifters who have been used to relying on force and body weight in order to transfer patients.

Manoeuvres for two operatives
The double blanket or carry sheet lift

Patients may be readily lifted by two lifters using a folded sheet or blanket. The blanket is folded in half and is placed under the patient to extend from behind his knees up to his shoulder blades. Once in position the lower ends are tied over the knees using a reef knot. The upper ends are gathered on either side to make a good hand hold and brought round under the axillae and held firmly in front. The lifters should then co-ordinate their actions to lift the patient off the chair using the power of their legs. (*See Figure 25.3*). The arms are kept straight throughout the lifting procedure. As soon as the patient's weight is off the chair the lifters come together to reduce the load distance factor.

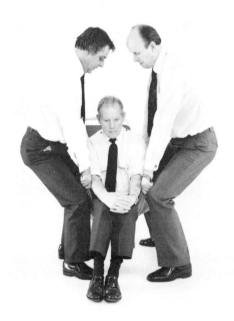

Figure 25.3 Double, blanket or carry sheet lift.

When placing the patient in his new location, a gentle swing action may assist in any increase in height that may be needed.

This technique may be utilized to raise a patient from the floor onto a chair. Foot positions are crucial in this manoeuvre.

Shoulder lift from the floor

This lift may be used to raise co-operative patients from the floor to a chair.

With the patient sitting with his legs in front of him, position the chair just behind him. Both lifters then kneel one on either side of the patient, the knee closest to the patient being level with his hip. Both lifters then put the leg furthest from the patient in a position as if preparing to stand up. The leg position then remains unaltered throughout the lift.

To locate the arm used in the lift (this is the arm closest to the patient) both lifters should sit back on the heel of the foot nearest to the patient, at the same time sliding the shoulder of the lifting arm under the patient's axilla.

If the lifters then pass the same hand and forearm under the patient's thigh as high up as possible, they link up with each other by means of a double or single wrist grip. After a final check, first of the chair position, and second that the patient's arms are properly located down the backs of the lifters, the manoeuvre is ready to commence (*see Figure 25.4*). Using their free hands, both lifters hold on to the side or the front of the chair onto which the patient is being transferred. On a count of three, the patient is raised by the lifters who straighten up into a kneeling position using the hip and buttock muscles as the power for the actual lift. The hand holding the chair can also provide some assistance in stability during the lift phase. Once the patient is level with the chair, he is located in the required position, before the lifters release themselves and stand up.

The Athlone floor to chair or bed lift

An alternative and generally more secure method of raising a seated patient from the floor to a higher level makes use of a folded carrying sheet, or folded blanket. This is located under the patient to extend from mid-thighs to the top of the lower back. The simplest method of locating the carry sheet is to ease the patient to one side so as to raise one buttock and thigh off the floor. The rolled carry sheet is then slid into position as far as it will go, and then the patient is gently eased onto the other side and the sheet pulled through.

The lifters take up a position on either side of the patient facing one another. The leading foot should be placed level with, or behind, the patient's hip, the other foot level with the patient's mid-thigh.

Squatting down, the lifters take a firm grip on the upper and lower edges of the carrying sheet or blanket. If carrying loops are fitted, these should be used. Both lifters ensure that their arms are kept straight throughout the lift, keeping a firm hold on the carry sheet, they stand up until the weight of the patient can just be felt as a slight

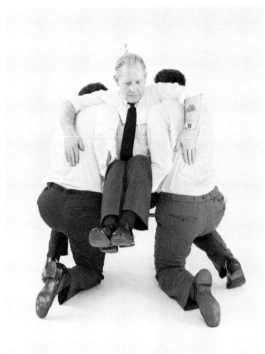

Figure 25.4 The shoulder lift from the floor.

resistance. After a final check that all is in order, both lifters stand up together using leg power to raise the patient up to the required level. By means of a gently swinging action, the patient is placed in the required position. The carry sheet may be removed in a similar way to the method used originally to place it under the patient.

The Athlone lift is particularly useful for patients who have only limited abilities and are therefore unable to co-operate. The security offered by the carry sheet and the fact that the patient can be observed throughout the manoeuvre are added advantages over the shoulder lift.

The six lifts detailed in this section are designed to illustrate how the transfer of patients can be achieved with minimal stress and maximum safety. Many variations of these techniques can be developed for use with specific cases and as long as the basic principles are adhered to, new lifts should be created when circumstances do not permit the use of the standard lifts. Ambulance personnel should check with their supervizors to be doubly sure that any new manoeuvre is safe and free from risk to the patient or themselves.

Lifting aids

The cot stretcher

When loading or unloading cot stretchers from ambulances the side lifting procedure should be used (*see Figure 25.5*). The stretcher should be placed close to the rear of the ambulance with the vehicle steps in a closed position. If the ambulance design will not allow the doors to open to 180 degrees place the stretcher far enough away to be sure that you are clear of the doors when lifting.

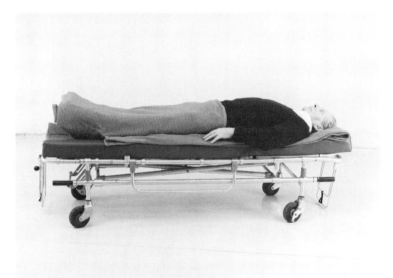

Figure 25.5 A blanketed patient on a cot stretcher in the lowered position.

The two persons position themselves, one either side of the stretcher facing each other. Place your hands palm upwards taking a firm grip of the lower rail of the cot frame (*see Figure 25.6*) below the patient's shoulders and mid-thigh levels, keeping your back straight, knees and hips bent and arms straight.

Adjust your hand position to compensate for any imbalance prior

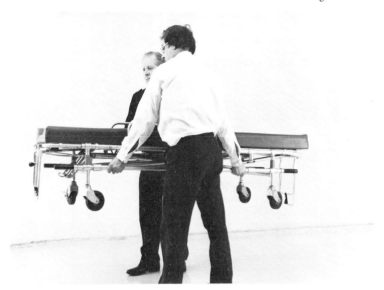

Figure 25.6 Loading a cot stretcher. Note that the hands are on the lower rail of the stretcher frame.

to the lifting. Keep your feet apart and pointing towards the ambulance.

Take a deep breath in, flex your arms keeping the back straight, and lift together keeping level to the full height necessary. Move in towards the stretcher to keep the weight close to your body.

Advance towards the ambulance placing the front stretcher wheels on the floor of the vehicle and feed the lower rail through your hands until all four wheels of the stretcher are on the floor. The stretcher is then carefully guided into its locking device so that it will be stabilized.

It must be remembered that lifting is only to be undertaken using the lower rail of the main frame. Under no circumstances is the stretcher to be lifted by the upper rail nearest the mattress. This technique can easily be mastered by people of varying height as when both are standing there is little if any difference between the distance from the ground to the knees. However, if this does constitute a problem, it can be compensated for by the taller person keeping the knees slightly flexed when lifting and/or positioning the hands further apart on the lower rail of the stretcher frame.

In order to unload, the reverse procedure is applied.

When using the York 4 stretcher, remember that it should never in the elevated position when loading or unloading, (*see Figure 25.7*), whilst being wheeled with a patient on, or whilst the ambulance is mobile.

Most conscious patients, given the opportunity, would prefer to travel facing the way the transport is going, thus the vast majority of cases may be loaded feet first.

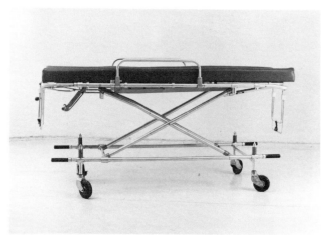

Figure 25.7 The stretcher in the elevated position.

The orthopaedic scoop stretcher

Place the stretcher alongside the casualty, (*see Figure 25.8*) so that you can adjust it to the required length, the patient's calves should rest on the lower plates, and the head on the upper plates. Turn the length adjusting pin (one either side, approximately one-third up from the foot of the stretcher) into the upward position which allows the stretcher to extend. There are four holes on each side of the tubular extending poles, and you should select the correct one and then turn the adjusting pins downwards into the locking position giving a slight tug to make sure all is well.

Uncouple the stretcher (*see Figure 25.9*) at its ends by pressing the coupling latch buttons which are found on the inside of both ends. Separate it into its two halves and place one on each side of the patient.

Kneel one on each side of the patient's body. One person should support the head, shoulders and pelvis and take up any slack in his clothing, whilst the other gently eases one half of the stretcher

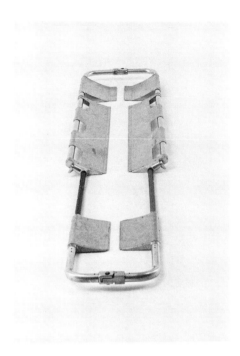

Figure 25.8 A scoop stretcher coupled together.

under the casualty, keeping it square. Repeat the procedure on the other side, taking care that the coupling latches are lining up and when you are satisfied that each side is correctly positioned, link both sides up again uniting the head end first. It is useful for one person to ease the pelvic area whilst the other couples the foot end into position.

This type of stretcher should only be lifted and carried by its end. It should not be held by the sides as this tends to spread the stretcher.

The patient is subsequently transferred to a conventional stretcher and the scoop stretcher removed. A canvas sheet should already be in position on the conventional stretcher so that any subsequent transfers which need to be undertaken can be made with the use of pole spreaders and stretcher canvas.

Uncoupling the scoop stretcher once it has been placed on a cot with the patient's weight on it sometimes causes difficulties, the simplest way to achieve success being to uncouple the foot-end latch and 'scissor' outwards and upwards lifting the head end clear.

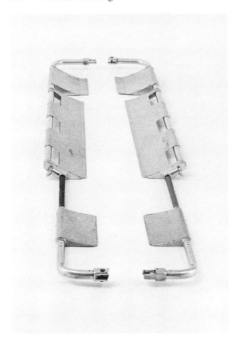

Figure 25.9 A scoop stretcher uncoupled.

It must be remembered that the scoop stretcher is an aid to lifting and is used as an alternative to the poles and canvas, etc. Straps are supplied to prevent unnecessary movement of the patient and to afford security when carrying them over rough ground or when negotiating a staircase. It is not a rescue stretcher and should not be used for this purpose.

Use of retaining straps

The stretcher has three retaining straps which are used when moving patients on the scoop out of difficult situations, (*see Figure 25.10*) or in confined spaces where it becomes necessary to turn a stretcher on its side, or even up-end it.

Strap No. 1
(1) The buckle is placed half-way across the chest.
(2) The running end of the strap goes across the chest, outside the upper part of the arms and into the side-hole of the stretcher. If

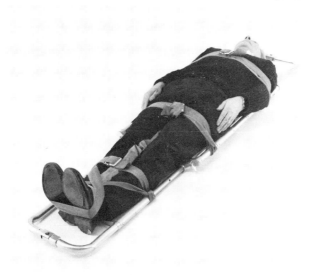

Figure 25.10 A patient attached to the stretcher via the three retaining straps.

this is pushed through about three or four inches it forms a loop, which the free end is then passed through (from foot-end to head-end) to form a half-hitch.
(3) Pass the free end back over the chest to the opposite side-hole of the stretcher, first around the bar and then back to couple up with the buckle in the middle of the chest. The strap is then tightened to the correct tension and any surplus is folded and placed as padding under the buckle.

Strap No. 2   Follow the same procedure that you have used for Strap No. 1, using side-hole No. 3, the strap running across the pelvis or upper parts of the thighs.

Strap No. 3
(1) The buckle is placed at the mid-tibial level.
(2) The running-end crosses the legs to the extension bar where a half-hitch is tied, pass the running-end across to the opposite foot to complete a figure-of-eight around the feet with a pad between the ankles, and the free-end around the opposite extension bar and back across the other leg to couple up with the buckle.

Securing a patient in the recovery position

Strap No. 1
(1) Place the buckle diagonally between the shoulder blades.
(2) The running-end of the strap goes diagonally up the back and over the collar bone. It needs to be padded and has to be held in position at this point by your partner until it has finally been tightened. Carry on with the running-end under the upper part of the chest to side-hole No. 1. Then secure with a half-hitch.
(3) The free-end is passed diagonally across the patient's back and into side-hole No. 2. and then up and diagonally across the patient's back to couple up with the buckle between the patient's shoulder blades. The strap is then tightened to the correct tension and any surplus is folded and placed as padding under the buckle. Your partner can now release his hold.

Strap No. 2   Repeat the procedure as for Strap No. 1, but on the other shoulder. The patient should appear as if he is in harness.

Strap No. 3
(1) Place the strap diagonally (face towards head, half way across the buttocks).
(2) The running-end of the strap goes diagonally across the buttocks into side-hole No. 3 and is secured with a half-hitch. A further portion of the running-end goes straight across the opposite side-hole and is secured with a further half-hitch.
(3) The free-end goes up on the same side as side-hole No. 2 to couple up with the buckle. Tighten straps to the correct tension and fold away any surplus. (Do not include hands or fingers in this strap).
(4) Pad well between the ankles and secure the foot to the lower side bars using a triangular bandage (*see Figure 25.11*).

A Paraguard stretcher

The Paraguard stretcher is a lightweight (22lbs) rescue stretcher which is safe and comfortable and which can be used for raising or lowering casualties in a horizontal or a vertical position (*see Figure 25.12*). It is contained in a canvas hold-all which can be easily carried on the back, or as a hand valise.

Use of the stretcher
(1) Unzip the cap of the bag by pulling on the two zips in opposite directions.

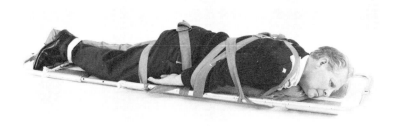

Figure 25.11 A patient attached to the stretcher in the recovery position.

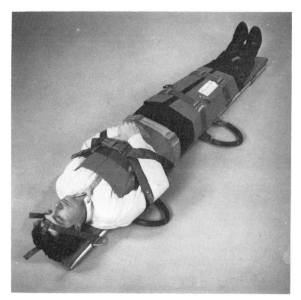

Figure 25.12 A patient attached to the Paraguard stretcher and ready for lifting.

(2) Invert the bag and the stretcher will drop out and automatically open with the back of the stretcher facing you.

(3) Lock the stretcher into one piece by turning and pushing forward the metal sleeves over the adjoining poles which lie one on each side to engage the bayonet lock, ensuring the spring loaded clip has risen through the hole.

(4) Unclip the carrying handle and any other additions as may be required to complete a particular operation, for example:
   (a) Lifting straps with rings which are found at each end of the stretcher.
   (b) A lifting sling for a horizontal lift (this is stowed in the pouch).
   (c) Fit the oxygen bottle under the straps provided at the head end.

(5) Turn the stretcher over and open out all the straps and corsets.

(6) Lay a canvas pole sheet on top of the grey pads. This will be used for transference at hospital, or if the Paraguard is required for more than one removal.

(7) Place the casualty on the stretcher with the head approximately one inch from the top end making sure there is good clearance of the axillae with the top part of the chest-corset.

(8) Fit the head-retaining strap and adjust for tension.

(9) Fit the chest-corset across the chest, leaving the arms out. Couple up the chest-restraining harness which is colour-coded (blue links with blue, yellow with yellow).

(10) Fit the leg corset around the lower limbs and couple up the leg-restraining harness (red to red and grey to grey).

(11) The feet-restraining harness (black) is placed around the instep of the feet in a figure-of-eight, and secured with the buckle opposite (also black).

(12) Elbow support harness. The casualties' arms are bent into a 'V' shape, the green elbow support harness is then brought over both upper limbs to secure them in the middle.

The buckles are of a special quick release type and are fitted with safety studs. Therefore, the hook must be coupled securely to the clip. Do not use inflatable splints where a Paraguard is to be used.

If the patient has to be raised or lowered in the horizontal position, either by ropes or helicopter winch, the four point lifting sling should be used. In the middle of the lifting sling is a metal ring to which the main rope or winch should be attached, running off the metal ring are two pairs of webbing straps, one short pair for attachment at the head end of the stretcher and a long pair for the foot end. These are marked on the inside of the strap, either head or foot. They are fitted with four metal 'D' rings which clip over the metal triangular lifting points found on the four side corners of the stretcher and are locked into position by turning the round nut on each. Guide ropes can be fitted to the rings of the lifting straps at the head and foot of the stretcher. For the patient who is being raised or lowered in the vertical position, attach a rope through the ring of the lifting strap at the head end of the stretcher. Two guide ropes should be attached to the carrying handles and this will avoid spinning and assist in the manoeuvre.

The use of canvasses in moving patients

A canvas sheet is approximately 2 metres (6 foot) long and 60 cm (2 foot) wide with 12 cm (5 inch) sleeves inserted on either side which take stretcher poles. Some types have no handles whilst others have handles on each corner.

Canvasses may be concertinaed width-ways or length-ways. In order to concertina a sheet width-ways, simply spread it out flat with the rough stitching side downwards, place your feet on one end of the sheet and pull it towards you making a fold every four to five inches, until you finish up with a pile of folds one on top of each other.

To concertina the sheet length-ways simply spread it out flat with the rough stitching side downwards and fold it length-ways in a 'Z' shape in three equal parts with the side edges facing opposite ways.

A sheet which is concertinaed width-ways may be used to move a patient who is in a supine or recovery position, or alternatively a patient in the sitting position.

Supine and recovery position

The concertinaed sheet is placed beside the patient in the hollow of the back (supine) or lower abdomen (recovery) with the upper end of the sheet pointing towards the head of the patient.

Method 1
(1) Whilst operator 1 stands astride the patient's pelvis, and using the clothing raises the patient slightly, the concertinaed sheet is passed through the hollow by operator 2.
(2) Select the number of folds you estimate it will take to reach the top of the head, and then operator 1 will stand on the rest. Operator 2 grasps the end of the sheet and pulls it upwards until the sheet reaches the top of the head whilst operator 1 steadies the body and shoulders.

(3) Operator 2 turns around facing the patient's feet and stands on the sheet just above the folds and holds the pelvis steady whilst operator 1 pulls the sheet, extending all the folds down to accommodate the lower limbs. The patient is now on a complete sheet.

Method 2

(1) Both operators kneel, one on either side of the patient's pelvis, and using the clothing raise the patient slightly. This should be done simultaneously and then the concertinaed sheet passed through the hollow.
(2) The operators select the number of folds necessary to reach the head and place their knees on the rest. The sheet is then pulled upwards together until the top of the patient's head is reached.
(3) Both operators simultaneously ease the rest of the sheet under the patient's buttocks and downwards to accommodate the lower limbs.

If you have reason to turn the patient such as may be necessary to put him in the recovery position, put a sheet alongside and turn the patient onto it.

Removal of a patient in the sitting position

This method is used for the removal of a patient who is in the sitting position such as in a car following a road traffic accident (RTA).

Use a sheet which has been concertinaed width-ways preferably one with handles.

The concertinaed sheet is slid down behind the patient as far as it will go with the end of the sheet which faces downwards lying nearest to the patient's body.

The end of the sheet which points upwards towards the head should be pulled up allowing about 5 cm (2 inches) to rise above the patient's head and this is then lifted over the seat. The operators position themselves one on each side of the patient and using the hand nearest the patient, grasp the clothing around the pelvic area (a belt or a pocket) and ease the patient upwards about an inch which should just be enough to allow the sheet to be slid down with the other hand. They should then pull the sheet downwards under the buttocks to accommodate the lower limbs, both working simultaneously. The patient can now be removed from the vehicle.

Snatch rescue

If a casualty has to be removed from beneath an obstacle such as a vehicle, first make a thorough assessment in order to ensure that nothing can trap the patient as he is being pulled free. Following this, a sheet which has been concertinaed width-ways, is placed under the patient's shoulders with the top end of the sheet facing the patient's head, the lower end facing the feet. The lower end is held firmly by someone placing a foot on each side of the bottom edge. The top edge is folded into the patient's clothing (the jacket or coat will do), the sheet and patient's clothing are then tightly grasped and traction is applied to slide both the sheet and the patient on it, out from beneath the obstacle. This should be done in one movement, once you have started keep going.

Uses of a blanket

Given ingenious improvization this simple piece of equipment can serve a variety of functions, for instance as a cushion, a pillow, a shawl or as a modesty covering. Here are a list of other suggested uses:

Coma roll

Take a full size blanket and fold into two unequal portions with the bottom end lying parallel to, but 30 cm (12 inches) below, the top end. Now fold this into quarters, *see Figure 25.13*. Roll this in from the side so that you have a thick roll and 30 cm (12 inch) long thinner roll. The thick part of the roll is placed under the patient's chest and abdomen whilst the thinner roll is passed under the patient's neck thus maintaining an open airway. It can be used for all unconscious patients placed in the three-quarter prone recovery position (*see Figure 25.14*).

Splinting

Take a full size blanket and roll it lengthwise as tightly as possible. This can then be used as an emergency splint for lower leg injuries (*see Figure 25.15*).

Padding

By folding or rolling a blanket you may be able to provide an adequate support for injured limbs which will make them more comfortable when being treated and transported.

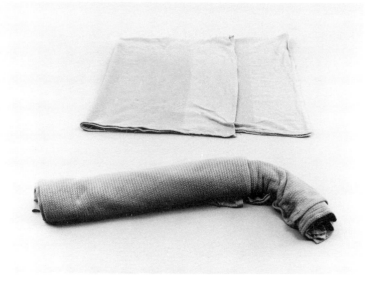

Figure 25.13 A blanket formed into a coma roll.

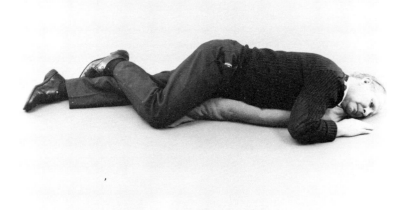

Figure 25.14 Patient in the three-quarters prone position with the coma roll *in situ*.

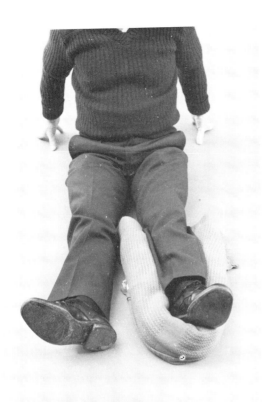

Figure 25.15 A blanket forming a temporary splint.

Resuscitation

Place a folded blanket under the back at the level of the scapulae and this will enable the head and neck to drop back into an ideal position for both exhaled air resuscitation and the Sylvester method (*see Figure 25.16*).

Spinal pads

Fold a blanket lengthwise into four then make 15 cm (6 inch) folds, approximately four are needed, from the bottom of the blanket to support the lumbar region and three from the top end to support the cervical spine (place the folds behind the nape of the neck as in *Figure 25.17*). This may of course be adjusted to fit the size of the patient.

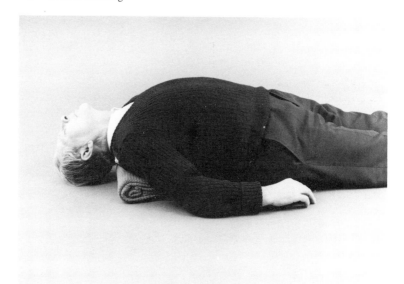

Figure 25.16 A folded blanket beneath the scapulae which, in this position, aids in maintaining an open airway.

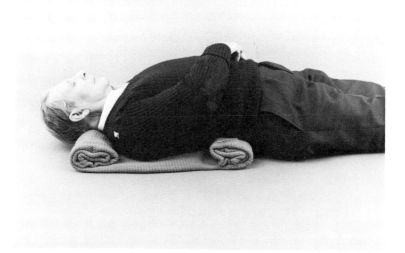

Figure 25.17 A blanket made up to form spinal pads.

Head stability

Fold the blanket lengthwise in four, roll tightly from each end, almost meeting in the middle, the head then being placed between the two rolls and held in position by a triangular bandage or frac-straps (*see Figure 19.7*).

Faciomaxillary injuries

Fold a blanket lengthwise into four and then fold each end towards the centre (using 15 cm (6 inch) folds) until the two piles of folds are about 20 cm (8 inches) apart. Repeat the procedure with another blanket and place it on top of the first blanket (*see Figure 25.18*). The patient's head is then positioned as shown, with a well beneath the facial bones, into which a small kidney dish may be placed to receive any blood, saliva or vomit draining from the patient.

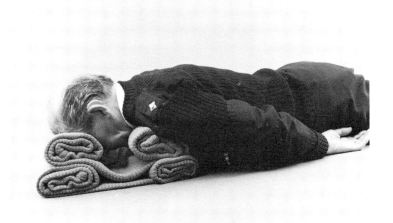

Figure 25.18 Two blankets used to support a patient with maxillo-facial injuries.

Cervical collar

Roll the blanket lengthwise and place around the patient's neck as illustrated in *Figure 25.19* to support the injured cervical spine.

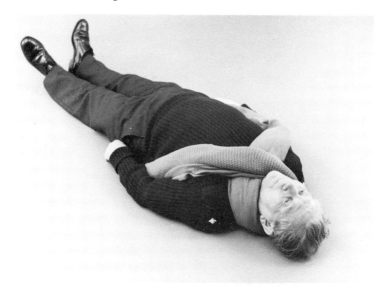

Figure 25.19 A blanket folded to form a cervical collar.

Use of a spinal board

Many of the injuries to the cervical spine that you will see will have occurred in RTAs. If such an injury is suspected the immobilization of the cervical and thoracic spines is paramount and a spinal board (*see Figure 25.20*) may be used to obtain this stability. Special care is required to extract a casualty from the vehicle in order that there should be no movement of the neck and although this procedure is often carried out unnecessarily it is vital that it is implemented whenever there is any suspicion of damage to the cervical spine.

(1) Instruct the casualty not to move and explain to him what you are going to do.
(2) Support the head and neck from behind, and maintain this support until the patient is safely secured to the spinal board.
(3) A cervical collar is placed under the patient's chin and around the neck (*see Figure 25.21*).
(4) Place the spinal board behind the patient's back. The easiest method is to insert the board from the side at an angle the top of the board first, with the rest of the board then slipped gently into position. If the patient has to be moved slightly forward to

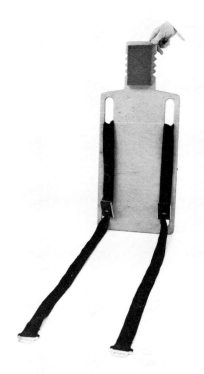

Figure 25.20 A spinal board.

accommodate the board, do this smoothly without jarring or twisting. The top of the board should be at approximately the same height as the top of the patient's head.

(5) Straps should be placed over the shoulders so that the buckles are resting on the abdomen, the bottom straps are placed over and down the inside of the casualty's thighs and brought up the outside of the thighs to couple up with the buckle of the opposite shoulder strap.

(6) The straps are now adjusted by pulling them together so that they are firmly in position diagonally across the chest.

(7) There will be a gap between the neck and the board, which must be padded before the head is tied with a restraining bandage.

(8) Immobilize the legs by padding and securing the ankles and

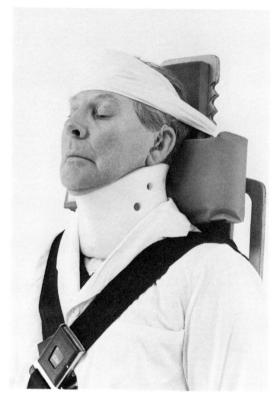

Figure 25.21 The patient now has his neck supported in a
cervical collar and his head firmly attached to the upper
portion of the board.

feet just above and below the knees with frac-straps or triangular bandages (*see Figure 25.22*).

(9) In order to extract the casualty without movement of the
board a concertinaed canvas sheet with handles must be used.

(10) After the sheet is in position and you have decided which way
the casualty is coming out, organize your helpers and position
your cot.

(11) Lift the casualty and board onto the canvas sheet and as soon
as possible lower the head of the sheet and raise the lower end
so that the casualty is in a lying position on the sheet. Gently
extract the casualty from the vehicle and place him on the cot.
Support must be given under the patient's knees by placing

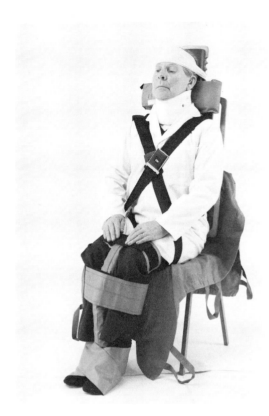

Figure 25.22 The patient is now ready for removal.

your arms there until the straps are released and then very gently, the lower limbs can be straightened.
(12) Secure the patient to the cot using the restraining straps, and load into the ambulance feet first.

Index